❋ ❙ ❋ ❙ ❋ ❙ ❋ ❙ ❋ ❙ ❋ ❙ ❋ ❙ ❋ ❙ ❋ ❙ ❋ ❙ ❋ ❙ ❋

Halt!

INSOMNIA

Simple Methods and Strategies to End Sleeping Disorder

❋ ❙ ❋ ❙ ❋ ❙ ❋ ❙ ❋ ❙ ❋ ❙ ❋ ❙ ❋ ❙ ❋ ❙ ❋ ❙ ❋

Cathrine Kowal

Table of Contents

Introduction

Insomnia… It is something that almost every single person on this planet will suffer from at one time or another in their lives and yet it is also something that most people know very little about.

It causes us to lay awake at night hoping for a little rest but never finding it. Left alone, it will only get worse and start to affect us in our everyday lives. It can affect our relationships, our jobs, and even our health. So, what should we do?

This book contains proven steps and strategies on how to end insomnia so that you can start getting the sleep that you need.

There are many causes of insomnia but one thing that remains the same in every case is the sufferers need to get a good night's rest. Insomnia can make us feel desperate, as if we are losing control of every area in our lives. It can make it very hard for us to understand and learn new concepts or just function in life.

That is why this book was created. No one should have to go to bed tonight knowing that they are not going to get the rest that they need. No one should have to get up in the morning exhausted from not being able to sleep the night before.

This book provides every remedy and technique that could be found to help treat your insomnia. From small changes that you can make to natural remedies and so much more, you are going to find everything that you need to know about treating your insomnia in this book.

It is important to me that you get the sleep that you need when you go to bed tonight and that is why I have put so much work into this book. I want to provide you with all of the answers to your questions and help you get the rest that you need.

As we work through each chapter of this book we are going to focus on the different tricks, tips, techniques, and remedies that you can use in order to treat your insomnia and finally get the sleep that you need.

These techniques, remedies, tips, and tricks are not only going to help you fall asleep faster, but they are also going to help you to stay asleep longer ensuring that your body is fully rested when you wake up each morning. You are going to be able to take on the world.

But for right now, let's worry about taking on that insomnia. Come on, let's get started right now so that when you go to bed tonight you will have the tools that you need to ensure you are able to fall asleep and wake up rested in the morning.

Chapter 1

What Is Insomnia?

Insomnia is a complicated sleep disorder that many people suffer from. Perhaps you are having trouble sleeping and have been wondering if you are suffering from insomnia.

According to the Mayo Clinic, insomnia is a sleep disorder that is very common. It makes it very hard for a person to fall asleep or to stay asleep. A person who is suffering from insomnia may wake up much earlier than they wanted to and find that they are not able to fall back to sleep. When a person who suffers from insomnia wakes up, they may not feel rested at all. Insomnia not only affects a person's sleep, but it can affect their quality of life, their performance at work, and even their health.

How Long Does It Last?

There are several different types of insomnia. The first one is acute insomnia. This means that it occurs for a short period of time and it is usually caused by something that is happening in a person's life. For example, when you cannot fall asleep because you are excited about something that is going to happen the next day. Or when you are so stressed out because of the way that things are going that you can't seem to sleep.

Each person is going to need a different amount of sleep, however, for most adults seven to eight hours per night should be fine. If you find that you need more sleep than this, you should talk to your doctor. If you are unable to get seven to eight hours of sleep each night because of an inability to sleep, don't worry, this book is going to help you catch some z's.

Most people will experience this type of insomnia at some point in their lives. The majority of people who suffer from acute insomnia are going to find that it passes on its own and does not need treatment.

Chronic insomnia on the other hand is when a person experiences insomnia no less than three nights each week for a duration of no less than three months. This insomnia usually needs to be treated in order to get the person back into normal sleeping patterns.

Comorbid insomnia is the type of insomnia that occurs alongside another medical condition such as depression or anxiety. Some of the medications that are used to treat certain conditions are going to cause insomnia. Those that are suffering from arthritis or severe back pain may have a hard time sleeping as well, which will cause them to suffer from insomnia.

Onset insomnia is what we call it when a person struggles to fall asleep.

Maintenance insomnia is the name for when a person has a hard time staying asleep. A person who has maintenance insomnia is going to wake up often during the night and will have a hard time going back to sleep.

In 2005 a study was done which found that 57 percent of women suffer from insomnia compared to 51 percent of men. According to this study, if you are a woman, you have a slightly higher risk of suffering from insomnia than a man. Sadly, only about 7 percent of people actually received treatment for their insomnia.

Women tend to suffer from insomnia more than men because of their hormonal changes. Insomnia can also be linked to depression in women. It is important if you think that you are suffering from depression that you seek professional help right away. You may find that with the treatment of the depression, your insomnia goes away.

One of the main reasons that women suffer from insomnia is because they give birth. Taking care of a new baby is very hard work and it would seem like a new mom would be able to fall asleep whenever the chance arose. Oddly enough, many new parents are struggling with insomnia.

It is likely that this insomnia is caused by the anxiety and stress that the parents have to deal with after their new baby's arrival. It is important however, for not just new parents but everyone to be able to learn the causes of their insomnia so that they can understand how to treat it best.

Think back to when insomnia started. Did something happen in your life that was traumatic at that time? Were you dealing with a lot of stress? Did a lot of changes happen all at once that you maybe were not prepared for? If you find that you can pinpoint a cause for insomnia, the chances are that it is acute, and it will go away once that problem that caused it is solved.

Learning how to spot the triggers for your insomnia is very important. Almost anything can trigger insomnia, so you need to make sure that you understand what is triggering yours. For example, if you are overwhelmed in your day to day life, spend a lot of time worrying about what is going to happen in the future, or are dealing with too much stimulation at one time, you may end up triggering insomnia.

Think about the days that have led to the nights that you were unable to sleep. What happened on those days? Where they particularly stressful? Was there something about them that made them different from the other days in your life? Make a note of any specific trigger that you find as you think about those days.

Start keeping track and look for triggers. When we do not sleep enough it can lead to insomnia getting worse. Part of this is because we are worried that we are never going to be able to sleep again, and part of it is because we dread going to bed at night knowing what a struggle it is going to be.

Try using a sleep journal. Write down what time you are getting up in the morning. Write down any naps that you take during the day and write down when you are going to bed at night. If you try to sleep and can't, write that down as well.

This is going to help you get an idea of how much you really are sleeping. Not too long ago, I had a woman come to me because she was unable to sleep at night. She talked about how she would lay in bed wanting to go to sleep but found herself unable to until the early morning hours.

I asked her to keep a sleep journal and what I found was that she was sleeping 4 to 6 hours per day. Because she was sleeping during the day when everyone was out of the house, she was unable to sleep at night. Once you reach those 8 hours of sleep, your body is not going to want to go to sleep. Sleep is not just a switch that you can flick and force your body into.

What had happened with this particular woman was that she had gotten so used to sleeping during the day that her body did not feel the need to sleep at night. She felt like she was suffering from insomnia because her body refused to sleep. I told her to stop taking naps during the day and she would be able to sleep at night. She didn't follow my advice because she was convinced that because she was not sleeping at night, she had insomnia.

Now I told that story to say this, I have found that a lot of the time, people are sleeping far more than what they believe, which leads them to think that they suffer from insomnia. Want a truly accurate reading of how much you are sleeping? Invest in a smartwatch and let it track your sleep patterns for a week. You may find that you are getting much more sleep or much less than you thought.

The reason that the woman in my story was unable to sleep is that she had messed up her sleep patterns. She had spent her time sleeping during the day instead of at night which caused her body to believe that daytime was sleeping time and nighttime was awake time.

Symptoms of Insomnia

When most people think about insomnia, they think about a person tossing and turning all night long unable to sleep. While insomnia does mean that you are not able to sleep at night there is much more to it. There are several different symptoms of insomnia.

- Difficulty sleeping is the number one symptom of insomnia. A person who has insomnia is going to have a hard time falling asleep or they are going to have a hard time staying asleep or both.

- Low energy levels or fatigue are other symptoms of insomnia. Feeling tired all of the time is something that most people with insomnia suffer from. When you are not getting enough sleep at night you are not going to feel energized the next day. Some people suffer from non-restorative sleep. This means that they do not remember waking up at night, however, they are still waking up tired in the morning. This could be a symptom of insomnia.

- Mood problems are another symptom of insomnia. If you feel irritable or as if you are in a bad mood all of the time with no identifiable reason it could be due to insomnia. When you do not get enough rest you can become aggressive, suffer from anxiety, or even become impulsive.

- Insomnia can lead to all sorts of relationship problems and I am not just talking about the relationship with your partner. You may find that you are having a hard time getting along with your family members, friends, or your coworkers. Remember insomnia can lead to mood problems which can affect our relationships.

- The inability to focus can also be a symptom of insomnia. When you are not getting enough rest, you may have a hard time focusing on your work. You may also find that you are making more mistakes or that you are missing deadlines. Insomnia can also lead to forgetfulness. While this is not your fault it is important to recognize that this is happening.

- When you are not getting enough sleep, you will find that you have a slower reaction time, especially when you are driving. This can put you at a very high risk of having an accident.

- Insomnia can lead to the development of other mental health disorders such as anxiety or depression. It can also lead to substance abuse because the person is so desperate to get some sleep.

- Those that suffer from insomnia can develop other health problems as well such as heart disease or high blood pressure.

- Not getting enough sleep can also affect your appearance. You may end up with dark circles under your eyes, puffy eyes, or a pale complexion. A lack of sleep can cause your body to retain water which leads to swelling.

- Hunger. When you are not getting enough sleep, your body begins interpreting hunger signals wrong. This can cause your cravings to be intense as well as out of control. Did you know that women who are sleeping less than five hours per night are more likely to become obese? The reason is that all of the crazy cravings they are dealing with due to lack of sleep.

- Insomnia can also lead to a weakened immune system. When you are not getting enough sleep, your body is more susceptible to viruses which causes you to get sick. Often this can lead to even less sleep than before.

- All of these symptoms can be caused by just missing a little sleep. Because when you suffer from insomnia, you are not getting much sleep at all, these symptoms can be much more intense.

Anyone can suffer from insomnia, however, there are some risk factors that you should be aware of.

1. If you are a woman you have a higher chance of suffering from insomnia. Some studies show that this could be due to hormonal shifts, menopause, or pregnancy.

2. Those that are over the age of 60 are at a greater risk of developing insomnia because as we age, our sleep patterns change. The older we get the higher our chances of developing insomnia are.

3. Certain mental disorders such as depression can cause insomnia as can any health condition in which you are prescribed a medicine that can affect sleep.

4. Those who are dealing with a lot of stress in their lives are at a greater risk of developing insomnia. If the stress is temporary, it is likely that insomnia will go away once the situation is handled. However, if you are under constant stress for a long period of time, you can develop chronic insomnia.

5. Anyone who does not follow a regular schedule can develop insomnia. For example, if you have to work swing shifts, if you travel a lot, or if you simply are not going to bed at or about the same time each night, you are at a higher risk of developing insomnia.

Of course, these are not the only things that can cause insomnia. Let's take a few moments and understand exactly what can cause a person to suffer from insomnia.

Chapter 2

What Causes Insomnia?

Sleep plays an important role in all of our lives. Without sleep we cannot feel happy, be healthy, succeed, or maintain any type of decent lifestyle. However, as many of us already know, sleep does not always come easily.

One of the main reasons that so many people are dealing with insomnia today is because of the increased amount of screen time that we all have. All screen time is included in this, such as when you are scrolling through social media, when you are watching television, playing a video game, surfing the internet, messaging your friends, or when you are doing research. Because we spend so much of our time in front of a screen it is important for us to understand what it is doing to us and how to ensure that it is not affecting our sleep.

What Is The Blue Light Effect?

Blue light is what we are naturally exposed to when we are out in the sun. While it is natural it does not mean that it does not come with side effects. These side effects can make it difficult for us to sleep at night.

Have you ever wondered why when you go out in the sun you feel so energized? It is because the blue light is what stops our bodies from producing melatonin. Melatonin is the hormone that our bodies produce to cause us to want to go to sleep. It also affects our circadian rhythm.

The circadian rhythm is nothing more than the clock that we have inside of our bodies that tells us when it is time for us to sleep and when it is time for us to wake up.

Every single device that we use that has a screen emits blue light. When we use these devices at nighttime, just before going to bed, or even while we are lying in bed waiting to go to sleep, our bodies are exposed to the blue light. Because the blue light stops the production of melatonin our bodies do not realize that it is time for us to go to bed. Our circadian rhythm gets disrupted and we end up suffering from insomnia. If we can fall asleep, we find that the quality of our sleep is not very good.

Using any device with a screen just 30 minutes before you go to bed can cause you to have problems falling asleep. Studies have found that using devices before bed can delay our REM sleep by at least another 30 minutes.

When you grab your device and head to bed, hoping that it will help you relax after a long hard day, you are actually telling your brain that you need to stay up longer.

Halt! **Insomnia**

Studies began as far back as the 50's on the effects of the blue light on our bodies, our sleep, and our circadian rhythm.

Even children who have televisions in their rooms can be affected by the blue light. Have you ever noticed that kids can stay up all night watching television without ever feeling tired? Or they can lay in bed on their phones until the wee hours of the morning? The reason is that as they are on these devices their bodies are not producing melatonin the way that they should be.

Spending time on our devices before we go to bed means that we are sleeping less and suffering from insomnia more. If you are suffering from insomnia the first thing that you should do is take a look at the amount of time that you are spending in front of a screen.

In order to get back on track the amount of time that we spend in front of a screen needs to be limited. While it is understandable that many of us have to use devices such as laptops in order to do our work, we need to do whatever we can to ensure that we are off of those devices no less than 30 minutes before we go to bed at night. Not only is this going to help you to fall asleep faster, but it is going to help you to get a better quality of sleep.

A great idea would be to set a limit on screen time to two hours before bed. You can do this for you and your children. You may want to remove all devices from the bedroom. No phones, no tablets, no computers, no televisions at all, at least in the evening time.

Our devices can provide us with a lot of benefits. They allow us to connect to the entire world, but they can also come with a lot of drawbacks. One of them is that they affect our sleep.

Stress

Stress makes our lives hard. It can make our lives even harder when stress starts to affect our sleep. Every person is going to respond differently to the stress that they have to deal with in their lives. Some people are going to sleep more when they are under a lot of stress, this could be due to depression or it could be that they are simply trying to avoid the stressor. More commonly, when people are under a lot of stress, they suffer from sleep deprivation due to stress.

When we are under a lot of stress, our bodies go into the fight or flight response. Our minds are constantly on alert. While our bodies know that we do need sleep our minds are so alert that they fight against the natural need for sleep.

On top of this when we are dealing with a lot of stress, the body releases cortisol into the blood. Cortisol is the stress hormone. Many people know cortisol as the hormone that makes us fat.

In a healthy person cortisol will begin to rise when they start to wake up in the morning. This is the time when the melatonin levels are at their lowest. By the end of the day, cortisol levels are dropping, and melatonin levels should begin rising in order to make you feel tired.

However, when you are under a lot of stress, your cortisol levels never drop. Instead they continue to stay elevated instead of dropping when it is time for you to go to sleep. This results in insomnia. A person who is under a lot of stress may struggle to fall asleep or they may struggle to stay asleep.

Stress in any area of our lives whether it be work, family stress, or mental illnesses can affect our sleep. Therefore, it is very important for us to learn how to handle the stress that we face in our lives.

So many of us try to take on everything at once instead of focusing on one thing at a time. This is one of the reasons that we are under so much stress. Instead, it is important that we focus on one task at a time. Trying to handle everything at once is going to cause your body to become overwhelmed and will send you right into the fight or flight response.

It also causes us to run around trying to put out fires instead of dealing with the problem before the fire starts. Focusing on reducing the stress in one area of your life is going to greatly improve your sleep quality. Once you have that one area managed you can continue to manage it while you begin to work on another area. Before you know it, you are going to see a huge reduction in the amount of stress that you have to deal with on a day to day basis and you are going to see your sleep improve drastically.

Constantly demanding yourself to do everything and to do it well is only going to lead to you becoming overwhelmed and overstressed.

Take time to enjoy life instead of constantly putting pressure on yourself.

Pain

Anyone that has suffered from any type of pain understands how hard it can be to get the proper amount of sleep. There are many disorders that can cause pain when we are lying down and it can cause us to have a hard time finding a pain free position to sleep in. Suffering from inflammation in the joints or from back pain is one of the most common pain complaints when it comes to insomnia. Of course, taking a pain reliever could help, however, it could also lead to dependence.

Try to find a position that does not cause you pain before you go to bed at night. For example, place a pillow between your knees in order to keep your hips aligned. Or if you sleep on your back place a few pillows under your knees in order to help reduce pain. Take an anti-inflammatory medication 20 minutes before you go to bed to help with any pain caused by inflammation.

If you are dealing with chronic pain, it is important for you to see a doctor. You have to be very careful when you are taking over the counter medications near bedtime because many of them contain caffeine or other stimulants that are going to make it very hard for you to fall asleep.

Caffeine

So many of us depend on caffeine to get us through our days. We live in a world where we are expected to be able to do everything, be everything, and never fail at anything. This causes many people to become dependent on caffeine. Whether it be in the form of energy drinks, coffee, soda, or energy pills, caffeine can cause a lot of health problems and of course it can make it difficult for us to sleep. Caffeine is addictive so reducing the amount of caffeine that you are taking in could be difficult. If you want to get a good night's sleep it may be necessary.

We use caffeine to keep us alert and awake and it is very good at its job. The problem with caffeine is when we are ingesting too much of it too late in the day. If you are ingesting caffeine after 2 pm you are going to find that you are having a very hard time falling asleep at night. The caffeine is still going to be in your system doing what it does best… Keeping you awake.

Paying attention to the amount of caffeine that we are ingesting each day is very important if you want to get a good night's sleep. The first thing that you need to do is stop ingesting caffeine at or before 2 PM. The later in the day that you ingest caffeine the harder it is going to be for you to fall asleep. If you can stop earlier than 2 PM, that is even better for your sleep.

This includes drinks such as tea or soda. Instead of drinking these with your dinner, or throughout the evening, drink some water instead. Trust me, your body is going to thank you for providing it with the water that it needs and giving it a break from all of the caffeine.

Of course, these are not the only things that can cause insomnia. However, they are the most common. As we continue through this book, we are going to cover some more reasons that you could be suffering from insomnia as well as how you can improve your sleep by using different methods and remedies.

Insomnia is going to be different in each person so do not feel as if there is no hope for you if you have not found an answer yet. We have much more to cover as we continue on, learning more about insomnia and how you can treat it.

Chapter 3

Side Effects of Insomnia

Every person on this planet is going to experience insomnia at some point in their lives. This is because there are so many things that can cause insomnia. Studies have shown that at least sixty million people deal with insomnia every year. They are waking up exhausted each morning and struggling throughout the day.

Understanding what happens when a person suffers from insomnia is very important. Many people try to suffer through insomnia hoping that it will go away on its own. While it is possible for acute insomnia to resolve on its own, it can still have many side effects.

1. Accidents- Having drivers on the road that are not getting enough sleep is hazardous not just for them but for the other people on the road. Being tired causes our reaction time to decrease when we are driving. It has been compared to driving while drunk. Each year 100,000 car accidents are caused due to drivers who are drowsy causing about 7,000 deaths.

Car accidents are not the only accidents that are caused by drowsiness. When a person is tired, they tend to get injured more at the workplace as well. It does not matter if they have done the job 1,000 times, if they are tired, they can easily make mistakes that they would not normally make, causing injury to themselves or others.

2. Cognitive Process- The cognitive process is also affected when a person does not get enough sleep. This means that our ability to think, learn, or process information is slowed down. Insomnia can make it hard for us to concentrate, can affect our alertness, and make it harder for us to solve problems. Lacking sleep causes the brain to not be able to function at full capacity, making it harder for us to complete everyday tasks or deal with even the smallest amount of stress. On top of all of this it can make a person very forgetful. They may forget important things such as appointments, deadlines, meetings, and even things as important as picking their kids up from practice.

3. Other Health Problems- Studies have shown that about 90% of those that have insomnia also have another health problem. These health problems can be caused by chronic insomnia. Health problems such as an irregular heartbeat, high blood pressure, stroke, or heart problems can all be a result of insomnia.

4. Mental Health Problems- It is not surprising that people who suffer from insomnia are five times more likely to

suffer from depression as well. Studies have shown that this depression can be caused by insomnia or it can be worsened by insomnia.

Insomnia and depression can cause a vicious cycle because of how they affect one another. Depression is worsened by insomnia and insomnia is often worsened by depression. As the cycle continues, they both continue to get worse. The good news is that most of the time if the insomnia is treated the depression usually gets better.

5. Premature Aging- Just one night of not sleeping enough can affect the way that we look. Missing just a couple of hours of sleep can cause our eyes to become swollen and dark circles to form. When we do not get enough sleep, our body produces too much cortisol which results in the collagen in our skin being destroyed. Collagen is what keeps our skin tight. When we sleep, hormones are released into the body to repair tissue. However, we a person does not get enough rest, this hormone is not released, and the tissue is never repaired which results in premature aging.

6. Life Expectancy Is Shortened- Those who suffer from persistent insomnia have a much higher risk of death than those who are sleeping 8 hours per night. Studies have shown that the risk of death can be increased by 97 percent compared to someone who does not suffer from insomnia.

There are many different reasons that the death rate is increased, however, the main reason is that the body is unable to properly function when a person is not getting enough rest.

When a person suffers from insomnia, they may spend a lot of time worrying about sleep or trying to sleep. This can actually cause insomnia to be worse because it increases the amount of cortisol or the stress hormone in the body. It is best to try not to worry about sleep but instead focus on relaxing in order to reduce the amount of cortisol in the body.

Chapter 4

Behavioral Changes

Understanding how your behaviors can affect your sleep may help you to understand what is causing your insomnia. You may also find that it is your thoughts that are causing you to have problems falling asleep or staying asleep. Cognitive-behavioral therapy is a program that many people use to make behavioral changes. Behavioral changes are beneficial to those that are struggling with insomnia because it allows you to deal with the actual problem that is causing you to have trouble sleeping instead of just taking a pill and going to sleep.

By identifying the thoughts and behaviors that are causing you to lose sleep, you can eliminate them or at the very least, learn how to deal with them. You can focus on these thoughts and behaviors on your own or you can have a therapist work with you.

The first thing that you are going to want to do is focus on using the bedroom for only sleeping and sex. This is not the place for you to do your work, play games on your devices, watch television or eat. When you go into your bedroom you are going to give yourself 20 minutes to fall asleep. If you do not fall asleep within that 20 minutes you are going to get back up and go do something else until you feel sleepy. When you begin to feel that you are ready to go to sleep you will go back into your room and try again giving yourself another 20 minutes to fall asleep.

Doing this is going to teach your body and your brain that the bedroom is for sleep and sex only. When you go into your bedroom your brain and body are going to respond by preparing for sleep.

It is also important for you to set a regular bedtime. This is often hard for adults to do. Many of us what to rebel a little bit and go to sleep whenever we decide to instead of at a specific bedtime. However, when you do not have a sleeping schedule your body has no idea when it is supposed to be tired. For example, if you stay up until midnight most nights playing games, how is your body supposed to know that you want to go to bed at 10 PM? You have to train your body to sleep when you want it to sleep.

This also means that you should not be taking naps during the day. When you take a nap during the day you are confusing your body. Of course, it is okay to take a nap if you are feeling under the weather, however, making a routine out of taking naps is going to affect how well you sleep at night. Your body is not only going to be confused about what time of the day you want to sleep but it is going to already be rested even if it is time for you to go to bed. This is going to cause your body to fight against going to sleep.

Do you find yourself lying in bed even when you are not tired? Just hanging out staring at the ceiling or texting your friends? Spending too much time in your bed can make it hard for you to sleep as well. Restrict the time that you are in your bed when you are sleeping or having sex. Again, this is going to teach your brain and your body that the bedroom is for sleeping and your brain as well as your body will begin to respond to that.

What do you do before you go to bed at night? Many of us are so busy that we do not stop until we hit the bed. We do not allow ourselves any time to wind down from all of the stress that we have to deal with each day.

While our to-do lists can seem to go on and on, we have to take the time to unplug as well as unwind before we go to bed each night. Unwinding before bed is going to help you get the rest that you need.

Give yourself 1 hour before you go to bed each night to allow yourself to wind down. It is understandable that an hour may be hard to carve out for some people however, given that you are going to benefit by finally getting the rest that you need, it will be worth it.

You can begin by taking a warm bath. One of the best ways for you to start winding down after a long day is to draw a warm bath. You can add bubbles, a bath bomb, bath salts, or essential oils. Using lavender scented anything is going to also help your body to relax. Light some candles to help set a relaxing mood.

As you are in the bath, allow yourself to fully focus on what you are doing. Focus on how the warm water feels on your body. How the soap feels against your skin. Experience all of the scents. Do not allow all of the stress of the day to fill your mind. Do not spend your time worrying about how much sleep you are going to get or all of the things that you need to get done.

Do not rush through your bath. Taking the time to enjoy the bath is going to allow your body to prepare for bed.

You can also prepare for the next day. You can write a list of all of the things that you need to do the next day. There are several different ways for you to do this. One is to simply write out a list of all of the things that you want to accomplish. The second way is to write out an hour by hour schedule and fill it in with the things that you want to get done. If you do this, you need to make sure that you are giving yourself enough time to get everything done.

You do not want to cause yourself more stress by overscheduling yourself. Don't try to fill your schedule with as much stuff as possible. Instead be realistic about the amount of time that each task is going to take you.

Deciding what clothes, you are going to wear the night before is also a great idea. When you know exactly what you are going to wear you are going to reduce the amount of stress that you have to deal with each morning. Prep your breakfast or at least know what you are going to eat. This will not only reduce the amount of stress that you have to deal with but it will ensure that even if you are running late you are able to grab your breakfast which will provide you with the energy that you need to get through your day.

Before you go to bed each night, sit down and write in a journal. You can write down the things that are bothering you and the problems that you are facing but don't forget to write down the things that you are thankful for as well. Writing down the problems that you are facing can help you to reduce the stress that you are dealing with because of them. Many times, it will also help you to find a solution to the problem.

When you take the time to practice gratitude and write down the things that you are thankful for or anything that made you happy each day, you are going to start to realize that things are not really as bad as you think they are. It is going to also allow you to go to bed at night with a positive mindset.

Using any of these techniques will help you to wind down before you go to bed at night. This will help you to relax and get the rest that your body desperately needs.

Many times, when a person is having a hard time sleeping it is because they feel that their life is out of control. You may feel like you are constantly busy, that you are not getting the things done that you need to get done, that your budget is out of control, and that you are failing all of the time.

When we feel that our lives are out of control, we are so focused on what is going on that our minds are working overtime, all of the time. When our minds are constantly going, we are unable to sleep because of all of the thoughts that we are bombarded with. Sound familiar?

If you are tired of dealing with a racing mind instead of getting the rest that you need, there are a few things that you can do in order to take control of your life back.

1. Decide what it is that you really want in your life and what you need. We are all wonderful at coming up with ideas when it comes to the things that we want. We want a bigger house, a newer car, a promotion, new clothes, the latest device, and the list could go on. What we have to do though is to decide what we really want. Happiness, peace, success, time to spend with our families… What is it that you really want?

   When you decide what you really want, you are going to be able to get there by setting goals and reaching them. Isn't this just going to create more for you to do? Not really. You see, as you are working toward your goals of creating the life that you want, you are going to be able to eliminate the things that do not support those goals. This is going to provide you with more time. When you are working toward the life that you want, you are going to find that you are more motivated to reach your goals and that your stress levels are reduced. This is going to lead to more peace of mind which will allow you to get the rest that you need.

2. Give yourself a little credit. We go through our lives, pushing ourselves to do more, take on more, and be more. When we have even the smallest failure we feel as if everything is falling apart. We have to give ourselves credit

for even our smallest accomplishments and stop focusing on our failures.

When we are focused on our failures, they can keep us up at night. We have to accept that everyone experiences failures, however, not everyone pushes themselves as hard as you do. Not everyone has seen the successes that you have seen in your life.

3. Take control of your budget. Are money troubles keeping you up at night? According to a recent survey money troubles are one of the main reasons that people are losing sleep. The survey showed that out of the 77 percent of people who lose sleep over something on their minds, 39 percent of them were worried about money.

Getting your finances in order may be exactly what you need to do in order to overcome your insomnia. The first thing that you are going to need to do is to check your credit score. Checking your credit score is not only about knowing what the numbers are but it is about finding out if there are any bills that you do not know about. Many times, I have heard about people checking their credit score only to find that they owe bills that they never received. Many of these are medical bills that were not sent to insurance companies; however, you may find something that you completely forgot about.

The next step is to create a budget. Write down all of your income and then write down all of the money that you have going out each month. Make sure that you include everything such as going out to eat, vet bills, entertainment, clothing, makeup, and anything else that you spend money on.

If you find that you are spending more than you are making you are going to have to start making some cuts. Look at where you could reduce your spending, habits you could stop, or ways that you could save money. Your goal should be to start a savings account, even if you are just putting 100 dollars per month into it, having it is going to help reduce your stress. You should also focus on paying off any debt that you have in order to reduce the amount of money that you have going out. Sure, you may have to make some cuts for a little while but knowing that your bills are going to be paid is going to help ensure that you are not staying up all not worrying about your finances.

4. What is the number one reason that people are losing sleep at night? Their relationships. This is not just their personal relationships, but it can be their relationships with their friends or their coworkers.

Think about the people that you spend the majority of your time with. Are your relationships with these people keeping you up at night? Perhaps the relationships with your children are causing you to lose sleep at night? Or the relationship with your partner?

The first thing that you need to determine is if the relationship is going to continue. If you are struggling with a relationship with a family member you may not have a choice but to continue the relationship however, unless it is a relationship with your children you may decide to step back from it a little bit.

Taking the time to think about what is going wrong in the relationship is a very important step. Journaling would come in handy at this point. When you journal, you are going to be able to write down what is going on in the relationship as well as how you are responding to it. You may find that you are overreacting. Or you may find that your relationship needs some work.

Is there a safe place that you have that will allow you to talk to the other person about your feelings and how the relationship is going? Being able to openly discuss the problems within the relationship is very important if you want the relationship to improve.

When you talk to the other person do not do so in an accusatory manner. Instead, focus on how you are feeling. Do not focus on what they are doing to make you feel that way but focus on what can be done to improve the relationship so that you can start getting some rest.

Take a look at how you are responding to the relationship. Are you getting emotionally worked up or acting out in anger? This is only going to cause more tension to build in the relationship. Take control of your emotions as well as your own behavior. Often, we find that it is our own behavior that is affecting the relationship that we are in and causing us to lose sleep.

5. Finally, stop making poor life choices. Stop accepting poor choices and poor behaviors in your life. Stop making excuses for the poor choices that you are making. When you make poor choices in your life you are going to have to live with the consequences which can weigh heavy on your mind. Of course, we are all going to make mistakes in life but simply accepting poor choices is different.

Think about the different areas of your life and how they are going. Do you find that there is one area or more than one area that you are always making poor choices in?

Each time you encounter a choice in your life you are going to have to make a decision. In order to make the best decision you need to take some time to determine what your options are, and which is best for you. While there are many choices that you can make that are not going to affect you in the long term, those that will, need to be thought out.

If you know that a decision is going to affect you in the future, take the time needed to ensure that you are making the best decision instead of just going with your emotions. For example, if you are in a relationship and you get into an argument you do not want to act in the heat of the moment and end the relationship. Your decision could last a lifetime and you could end up regretting it. Instead, take the time to think about the consequences of your decision and to determine if it is really what you want to do. Then make the decision.

We have to remember that every area of our lives can affect our sleep and when we are having problems in any area, it can lead to insomnia. This is why it is important to not just focus on getting enough sleep but to ensure that every area of our lives gets the attention that they need.

Chapter 5

What's A Pink Elephant?

What is a pink elephant? Don't think about the pink elephant. We have talked a lot about how focusing on different areas or worrying about different things in our lives can cause us to suffer from insomnia. We have also talked about how it is important to not focus on these things when we are trying to fall asleep.

Still thinking about that pink elephant? This is known as the pink elephant effect. When we are told not to think about something, we cannot help but think about it. The same goes for when we are trying to go to sleep. When we know that we should not be focusing on something that is exactly what we end up thinking about.

Imagine that you are stressed out about something that is happening at work. It is after midnight and all you want to do is fall asleep. However, that simple mistake that you made yesterday at the meeting keeps popping into your mind or you find yourself worrying about an offhanded remark that your boss made. You lay there telling yourself that you have to stop thinking about it and that you have to go to sleep but that only makes you think about it more.

This causes you to become more distressed and causes it to be harder for you to fall asleep.

This is exactly what the pink elephant effect is. In order to stop yourself from thinking about whatever your pink elephant is, you may try to distract yourself and think about something else, but you will find that the pink elephant keeps popping into your head. The harder you try to not think about the pink elephant the more you focus on it.

So how can you stop thinking about the pink elephant? Well, you can't. Instead, you have to accept that you think about it. "Yes, I have thought about the pink elephant. It does exist. And if I think about it that is okay."

When you decide to stop struggling against your own mind you will find that whatever your pink elephant is, begins to leave you alone and you're able to get to sleep faster.

Telling yourself that you cannot think about a specific thing is only going to cause you to think about it more. Therefore, you need to accept the thought as it comes into your head and allow it to pass.

Deep Breathing Exercises

If you are still unable to clear your mind you may want to try some deep breathing exercises in order to help you get to sleep and stay asleep. Deep breathing exercises are a great way for you to take your focus off of everything except for your breathing which will allow you to fall asleep and help you to overcome your insomnia.

As you are lying in bed, close your eyes and blow all of the air out of your lungs through your mouth. Take a deep breath through your nose as you count to 4 in your mind. Hold that breath for 7 seconds. Blow all of the air out of your lungs as you count to 8. Repeat.

You will continue to do this focusing completely on your breathing as you lie in your bed. You will begin to feel your body relaxing as you continue this breathing exercise and before you know it, you are going to find that you are falling right to sleep without thinking about any of the troubles that normally keep you awake at night.

Deep breathing is one of the best methods of reducing insomnia because it allows the body to begin to relax and it helps to quiet thoughts. Some have found that by using techniques such as this one, they are able to fall asleep within just 60 seconds.

You can also use some of the techniques that we talked about earlier in this book to calm your mind and prepare it for sleep. Using a bedtime routine is going to help your body to understand when it is time for you to begin winding down and getting ready for rest.

Meditation

Meditation is a great way to help your body relax before bed as well. You do not have to have any experience in meditation in order to use it. Meditation just like deep breathing helps the body to relax. It allows you to clear your mind so that you can get to sleep quickly.

Halt! **Insomnia**

There are many different types of meditation that you can use. However, one of the easiest ways for you to meditate is to use a guided meditation. Choose a guided meditation that you can find online and begin playing it as you wind down for bed. If necessary, you can place your device across the room as you allow the meditation to play. You can even listen to it as you soak in a warm bath before bed.

When you lay down, continue listening to the guided meditation as you prepare to fall asleep. You can continue to allow the guided meditation to play as you sleep. It is going to work with your subconscious to help you get a better night's rest.

You may find that while you are listening to the guided meditation that thoughts try to enter your mind. Instead of focusing on these thoughts, you will simply acknowledge them and let them pass.

Do not allow yourself to focus on the thoughts as they enter your mind. Do not allow worries to take your focus off of the meditation. If you find that you are having a hard time not focusing on the thoughts that enter your mind, focus on your breathing.

Simply focus on inhaling and exhaling as your mind clears and your body starts to relax.

Continuing to use meditation is going to help reduce insomnia over time. Your subconscious is going to be rewired to sleep when you are in bed as you continue to listen to the meditation as you sleep.

If meditation just isn't your thing, try listening to some relaxing music as you fall asleep. Classical music has been proven to help people fall asleep and stay asleep. This is going to help you get a better night's sleep as well.

Mindfulness

What is mindfulness? Mindfulness means that we are fully present and aware of whatever it is that we are doing. If for example, you are taking a shower, you are focused completely on the act of taking a shower. You focus on the smell of the soap that you are using, how the water feels when it hits your skin, and how the bubbles feel as they roll down your body.

When you are mindful, you do not spend your time worrying about what has happened in the past or what is going to happen in the future. Instead, you understand that this moment that you are experiencing is never going to happen again. You are never going to be doing what you are doing in this exact moment ever again. Sure, you will take another shower, but it will be in another moment. A moment that you will be mindful of.

Because our lives are so over-scheduled, because we have so much to do and so much stress in our lives, we spend a lot of our time worrying about the things that have happened in the past and the things that may happen in the future. We are constantly worrying about the situations that are going on in our lives, about the people that are in our lives, our jobs, our finances, and so on.

By choosing to practice mindfulness we are able to take a step back from all of the stressful situations in our lives. Instead of focusing on all of our worries we choose to experience every single moment in our lives.

Practicing mindfulness in every area of our lives is important. When we are at work, we should be mindful of the work that we are doing. We should be completely focused on the work that we are doing, choosing not to focus on any trouble we are experiencing at home, or in other relationships in our lives. When we are at home, we choose to experience those moments instead of focusing on or worrying about any problems that we are facing at work.

When we are eating our meals, we are completely focused on the food, the tastes, and the smells instead of checking our emails or scrolling through social media.

Of course, when we go to bed, we are completely focused on the act of resting instead of worrying about all of the troubles that we deal with during the day.

Studies have shown that mindfulness can help to reduce sleep disorders. Practicing mindfulness is a great alternative to medications and it should be something that you try before taking any sleeping pills.

Start by using mindfulness in your everyday life. Focus on being fully present in each moment of your life. Mindfulness can reduce insomnia that you suffer from, but it can also improve the quality of your sleep, increase the amount of time that you spend sleeping and make your sleep more effective. This means that you will feel rested when you wake up in the morning.

How can you practice mindfulness? Simply focus on whatever it is that you are doing. If you find your mind wandering simply bring it back to what you are doing. Use all of your senses no matter what it is that you are doing. Notice the sounds around you, the smells, the tastes, the feeling of whatever is in your hands, and all of the colors that surround you. Using all of your senses is going to help you focus on what you are doing and fully experience the moment.

Positive Thinking

Many people who struggle with insomnia live in a state of denial. They tell themselves that they will be asleep soon or that they will sleep tonight even though they have not slept in three nights. They stare at the clock, "If I fall asleep right now, I will still get three hours of sleep." As the clock continues to tick, they continue to count the number of hours of sleep that they will get if they fall asleep right at that moment.

Counting down the number of hours that you have left before you have to get out of bed can cause a lot of anxiety. Instead, of focusing on the negative, focusing on the positive will lead to more sleep. Lying in bed and accepting that you are still awake but not worrying about it will reduce the amount of anxiety that you have to deal with.

Instead of focusing on how few hours you have to sleep, try thinking about how much you are sleeping each night. Use your smartwatch to track the number of hours that you are sleeping each night. You may find that you are getting more sleep than you thought. While this may not be the amount of sleep that you need, at least you are getting some sleep.

Positive thinking means that you are taking responsibility for the way that you think about the things that happen in your life. You have a choice as to how you react to whatever is going on in your life including your lack of sleep.

Thinking positively about whatever is going on in your life is going to help you reduce the amount of worry that you have to deal with. When you choose to think positively about every situation in your life you are going to be able to shift your negative mind frame and feel better about your life in general.

In order to think positively you have to take responsibility for your thoughts. You are the only person that is in control of your thoughts. You can choose to focus on the negative and have a negative mindset, causing yourself more anxiety than necessary or you can choose to have a positive attitude and create a positive mindset.

In order to change your mindset, you need to understand the benefits of positive thinking.

Positive thinking can add years to your life, it reduces distress in your life and can even help with depression. When you think positively you are less likely to develop a cold and you tend to be healthier both mentally and physically. When you do have to deal with stress, you are better able to cope with it and that is what causes positive thinking to help with insomnia.

One of the hardest parts of positive thinking is reducing negative thinking. In order to reduce your negative thinking, you have to learn how to identify those negative thoughts.

For example, "If I don't fall asleep right now, I'm not going to get any sleep and I am going to have a terrible day tomorrow. I am not going to be able to focus on anything and my boss is going to get mad."

When thoughts like this enter your head, you have to identify them and replace them with more positive thoughts, "I may not be falling asleep as fast as I would like but I am still going to get some sleep. Some sleep is better than no sleep and even if I don't get enough sleep, I am going to be able to do everything that I need to get done."

You can write the negative thoughts down that you have on a regular basis and then write down something that you can tell yourself instead, such as the example above.

Then think about all that you have accomplished at work without getting the proper amount of sleep. The chances are that if you have had all of those accomplishments while not getting enough sleep you can get through one more day.

How is this going to help insomnia? When you stop focusing on your lack of sleep you will increase your chances of actually falling asleep. Remember when we talked about clearing your mind and the pink elephant? Focusing on falling asleep can be your pink elephant. While your mind is trying to figure out how many hours of sleep you would get if you fell asleep at any given moment you are allowing your mind to keep you awake.

Choosing not to think negatively about your insomnia is going to allow your mind to be cleared which will lead to you falling asleep.

Chapter 6

Is It What You're Eating?

Have you ever found yourself lying in bed at night staring at the clock and wondering what is wrong with you? Why can you not ever seem to fall asleep? It could have something to do with what you are eating. What you are eating can affect your sleep and can cause you to suffer from insomnia.

We already know how important sleep is to our bodies and to our lives. Most people today try to delay going to sleep as much as they can. Even if they want to get more sleep, they may be doing things that are causing it to be harder for them to get the sleep that they need.

Certain foods that we eat have the ability to interfere with our sleep and can even cause insomnia. Of course, the most obvious thing that we consume which is going to keep us awake is caffeine, however, there are plenty of other foods that can cause it to be hard for you to get the rest that you need.

Fried foods take a long time for your body to digest because of the high-fat content which makes it hard for your body to get the rest that it needs.

Beans are another food that is hard for the body to digest. While beans are very good for you, the body has to work a long time to digest them and this can interfere with your sleep. Another reason that they can interfere with your sleep is that they cause gas which can be painful.

If you suffer from heartburn when you eat spicy foods, they could lead to insomnia as well. When you are suffering from heartburn it can be very difficult to fall asleep, especially if you sleep on your back which causes heartburn to become more noticeable.

Foods such as broccoli that are high in fiber can make it harder for you to sleep. Again, these foods take a very long time for your body to digest which causes it to be hard for your body to rest.

Eating an unhealthy diet can also lead to insomnia. Prepackaged, processed foods are filled with fat and sugar which are going to make it hard for you to get the sleep that you need. Not only are they not good for your sleep but they are not good for you in general. When you do not take care of your body you cannot expect it to work properly. That is why it is very important for you to make sure that you are eating a healthy diet.

Changes You Can Make

The first thing that you are going to want to do is to pay attention to when you are eating. Eating less than 3 hours before you go to bed at night can cause you to have a hard time going to sleep because your body is trying to digest the food that you ate.

While eating and then going right to bed is not technically bad for you and it is not going to make you gain weight if you are eating healthy foods, it can keep you up late into the night.

Make sure that you are not drinking alcoholic beverages before going to bed. Sure, it may seem like alcoholic beverages are helping you to sleep but when you drink in order to sleep you are not getting into REM sleep which is what you need in order to concentrate, learn, and do almost everything that you need to do. It is during REM sleep that your body gets the rest that it needs.

Do not eat large meals. Large meals take longer to digest. Instead of eating large meals throughout the day, choose to eat more frequent smaller meals that will take less time for your body to digest.

Changing Your Eating Habits

Studies have shown that a high sugar, high saturated fat, low fiber diet causes insomnia. Of course, most of us know that if we eat a diet that is high in sugar as well as saturated fats while being low in fiber, we are going to suffer all sorts of health problems and likely become fat. This can make insomnia even worse.

Knowing that our food choices affect our sleep simply is not enough though. We have to choose to change the way that we are eating not only to improve our quality of sleep but to improve our overall health as well.

If you are suffering from insomnia it is likely that you are finding it hard to control your weight. This is because insomnia often leads to weight gain. By taking control of what you are eating therefore reducing your insomnia you will also find that you are going to start losing weight.

Studies have shown that when a person eats a high fiber diet they are going to sleep better and deeper than those that eat a diet that is high in saturated fats, sugars, or other carbs.

You don't have to become a super picky eater in order to change your eating habits so that you can sleep better. (Bringing your own dressings when you go out to eat or not being able to order anything off of restaurant menus). Simply making some better choices is going to help you to not only sleep better but to improve your overall health.

I'm not talking about going to the extreme here and overhauling your entire life. Instead, I am talking about making some small changes that will provide you with big results.

Studies have actually shown that when you make small changes, focusing on one habit at a time you are going to have more success than you would if you tried to overhaul your entire diet.

Along with changing some of your old eating habits in order to improve your sleep, you can add some new healthier habits as well. So, here are some changes that you can make to your diet that are going to improve your eating habits in order to help you sleep better.

1. Start adding frozen vegetables to everything that you cook. Frozen vegetables are a great choice when it comes to getting in the veggies that you need. Frozen vegetables are frozen in a way that ensures that they keep all of their vitamins and nutrients. Adding them to the meals that you are already cooking such as omelets or kinds of pasta will help you boost the nutritional value of the dishes and ensure you are getting all of the fiber that you need.

2. Go grocery shopping once per week. Going grocery shopping is something all of us would rather not do but when we take the time to go to the grocery store and get all of the ingredients that we need so that we can cook our food at home, we are less likely to end up going out to eat. Make sure that you prepare a meal plan ahead of time so that you know what ingredients you are going to need and make a list. Stick to that grocery list when you are shopping. It is so easy for us to see all of the delicious looking prepackaged foods at the grocery store and want to add them to our cart. We have to remind ourselves that those foods could affect how much we are sleeping and right now, sleep is much more important.

3. When you make your plate split it up into three sections. Fill it with ¼ complex carbohydrates, ¼ of any protein, and ½ of vegetables. This will ensure that you are getting all of the nutrients that your body needs and that you are eating a balanced diet.

4. As we sit down to eat it can be tempting to dig into the carbohydrates first but be mindful of what you are doing. Instead, start with your vegetables, eat all of them first and then move on to your protein. Save your carbohydrates for last. When you do this, you are not going to be as hungry when you get to the carbohydrates and may find that you don't need them as much as you thought you did. Of course, if you are eating healthy complex carbohydrates, if you want to eat them that is perfectly fine as well. These would include brown rice, whole grain pasta, multi-grain bread, and other foods that are made out of whole grains.

5. Make an extra serving of protein each night so that you can toss it into a salad to eat for lunch the next day. This is going to help ensure that you do not make a fast-food run when you get hungry but instead, your healthy delicious salad will be right there waiting for you.

6. If you are going to have coffee in the morning, use unsweetened almond milk instead of creamer or regular milk and sweeten it with your favorite sweetener instead of sugar. The less sugar you have in your diet, the more likely you will be able to fall asleep faster and stay asleep longer at night.

6. Eat a healthy breakfast that is high in protein and vegetables. It is very tempting for us to grab a sweet sugary breakfast. We have so many choices when it comes to donuts, croissants, and even sugary cereals but if you want to sleep better at night, focus on the protein and vegetables.

7. Choose to drink water. Your body needs water. No matter how much you want to fight against that fact, it remains true. Choosing to drink water, at least in the afternoon is going to allow your body to not only become hydrated but get rid of all of the caffeine that has been pumped into it through coffee and other sugary drinks that we all turn to each day. Avoid energy drinks as well. I understand that this may be hard because you are tired and just trying to stay awake but the energy drinks are going to affect your sleep and you are going to find yourself caught in a vicious cycle of energy drinks, insomnia, and more energy drinks.

8. If you have the choice, pick whole foods instead of processed foods. There are going to be times when you do not have a choice about what you are eating, especially if you are eating at work. However, when you do have the choice, choosing whole foods is going to help you get the rest you need at night and it is going to help improve your overall health.

9. Speaking of work, bring food with you to work or wherever you go. Go out and grab some food storage containers for your leftovers, snacks, and your lunches. When you cook dinner at night, make sure that you are cooking enough for you to take to

work the next day. At the very least, pack your lunch and snacks for the next day before you go to bed at night so that you are not tempted to eat junk and affect your sleep.

10. Write down all of the food that you are eating every day for one week. Most of us eat a lot more than we think that we do. We also eat a lot more, unhealthy foods than we think that we do. Take one week and write down all of the foods that you eat in order to get a better idea of your eating habits as well as how much food you are eating. You can also write down how you are sleeping each night and see if the foods that you are eating correlate to insomnia that you are suffering from.

11. Before you go back for seconds give yourself 20 minutes. Your stomach takes 20 minutes after it is full of telling your brain that it is full. We can all heat our food up if we decide that we need it later. Eat a normal portion of food at your meals and then wait 20 minutes. If you do decide to go back, make sure that you go back for vegetables for that second helping. Vegetables are low in calories and they are high in fiber which is going to provide your body with a lot of nutrients while ensuring that the food that you are eating does not affect your sleep.

Making small changes to your diet is going to make it easier for you to sleep at night and it is going to improve your overall health which is actually going to continue to improve your sleep.

Foods That Make You Sleep Better

There are certain foods that you can eat in order to improve your sleep. These foods are going to cause your body to release certain hormones that help to induce sleep.

These foods are going to help your body to increase the amount of serotonin and melatonin that your body is producing before you go to bed. On top of this, some of them are going to contain zinc, magnesium, and calcium which are also going to help you get more sleep.

Eating these foods close to bedtime, just before that one hour of wind downtime that we talked about earlier in this book, is going to help your body prepare for bed. It is important, however, to make sure that these foods do fit into your daily calorie count to ensure that you are not overeating and gaining weight which is going to cause you to have more sleeping issues.

We have all heard the stories of drinking warm milk before going to bed in order to sleep better and studies have shown that there may be something to this. Warm milk helps to increase the amount of melatonin that your body produces and because it has calcium as well as other vitamins and minerals that will help induce sleep.

Tart cherries are one of the best ways for you to get some extra melatonin naturally. You can choose fresh cherries, dried, or frozen. You may also drink some tart cherry juice in order to help induce sleep.

Halt! **Insomnia**

Any food that contains tryptophan is going to help induce sleep as well. Most of us have heard of the effects of tryptophan because of the effect that turkey has on us on Thanksgiving Day. We know that when we eat turkey, we suddenly feel tired and want to head straight to bed. Any food that contains tryptophan is going to have the same effect on your body. These foods include red meat, eggs, oats, turkey, tuna, bananas, milk, and even peanuts.

Foods that help to increase serotonin in the brain are also going to help you to fall asleep faster and stay asleep longer. Studies have shown that these foods help to regulate the wake-sleep cycle and they help us to have a better quality of sleep.

Complex carbohydrates are going to help to increase the amount of serotonin in the brain. These foods include, nuts, oats as well as other whole grains, and fruit. Avoid any food that contains caffeine because caffeine suppresses the serotonin levels in the brain.

Not only are these foods going to help increase serotonin but many of them help to increase the levels of melatonin in the body. This means that while the foods are going to help you feel at peace and relaxed, they are going to help induce sleep as well.

Kiwi is a great fruit for you to eat if you want to get a good night's sleep. Eat just 2 kiwis 1 hour before you go to bed. You can do this during your wind downtime. Studies have shown that when you eat 2 kiwis 1 hour before you go to bed at night you are going to sleep longer and with fewer interruptions. On top of that kiwi fruit has been shown to prevent depression.

If you are really having a hard time sleeping vitamin D or the lack of it might just be the reason. So many of us are lacking in vitamin D because a lot of our jobs force us to spend all of our time inside. Vitamin D is the vitamin that we get from spending time in the sun. Because we are inside so much our bodies simply are not producing it and that is affecting our sleep.

You can find vitamin D in tuna, salmon, sardines, and mackerel. If you can't stomach these foods, don't worry. You can take a multivitamin that contains vitamin D, or you can take a vitamin D supplement. If you do choose to take vitamins or a supplement, make sure that it is a quality brand. Many brands have been proven to not contain any of the vitamins that they claim to contain. Talk to your doctor about the best brands available to you or at the very least, talk to your pharmacist. While these vitamins and supplements may cost a little bit more, they are going to provide you with what you need instead of leaving you hanging and that means that you are going to start sleeping better.

Omega 3-Fatty Acid has also been proven to help improve the quality of your sleep. You will get Omega 3-Fatty Acids from fish such as salmon and tuna. Studies have shown that not only are these going to help improve the quality of your sleep, but they are also going to help manage depression.

Of course, you can take an Omega 3-Fatty Acid supplement but as I already said, make sure that you are purchasing a high-quality supplement. You do not want to waste your money on a supplement that does not contain any Omega 3-Fatty Acids and a low-quality supplement is not going to help you get the sleep that you need.

Any food that contains zinc or magnesium is going to help you get the sleep that you need. Both zinc and magnesium have a direct effect on the melatonin levels in your body. There have been studies that have shown that when a person takes a supplement containing magnesium and zinc, their insomnia improves drastically.

You do not have to take a supplement though. You can get the zinc and the magnesium that you need from the foods that you eat. You can get more magnesium in your diet by eating more seeds and nuts, legumes, dark leafy greens, fish, avocado, whole grains, dried fruit, bananas, and even dark chocolate.

If you want to get more zinc in your diet, you will want to add in extra nuts and seeds, dairy products, beef or lamb, and beans.

Herbal teas are a great item to add to your diets in order to help you fall asleep at night. It is important when you are adding herbal teas to your diet that you make sure that they do not contain any caffeine. Try drinking some chamomile tea as you wind down for bed at night. Drinking a cup of chamomile tea sweetened with honey or your favorite alternative sweetener is going to help you to relax and fall asleep faster. Try drinking a cup of tea as you soak in your warm bath at night.

Making these small changes are going to help you to improve the quality of your sleep as well as the amount of sleep that you are getting each night. Many of these changes are also going to help to improve your overall health as well. You may find that once your health starts improving your quality of sleep starts improving as well.

Don't feel as if you have to make all of these changes all at once. Instead, pick a couple of changes that you want to start working on and focus on these. As you start to see improvements in your health and your quality of sleep, you can start making more changes. As long as you stay committed to these changes your sleep is going to improve.

Chapter 7

Stress Can
Cause Many Sleep Issues

❀ ❀ ❀ ❀ ❀ ❀ ❀ ❀ ❀ ❀ ❀ ❀ ❀

Stress is a huge factor when it comes to insomnia. Stress can make it hard for us to fall asleep at night and it can make it very hard for us to stay asleep if we are able to fall asleep.

Every person is going to react to stress differently. Some people may end up sleeping all of the time when they are dealing with a lot of stress. This is because they are trying to avoid their problems by simply avoiding what is making them feel stressed. Other people are going to have a hard time falling asleep because the only thing that they can think about is their problems. They may end up overthinking whatever is causing them stress which is only going to cause them to have to deal with more stress.

Stress causes us to go into the fight or flight response. Our bodies and minds become hypervigilant or always on alert. This causes us to not be able to relax. When we go into the fight or flight response, our body responds by releasing cortisol. As we already learned in this book, cortisol is known as the stress hormone. Too much cortisol in the body can do a lot of damage.

Because cortisol levels remain high all of the time instead of lowering at night as they are supposed to, we find that we are unable to sleep.

Stress Management

When we are dealing with a lot of stress, it can seem as if we have no control over the situation. This is what leads us to feel overwhelmed and causes us to suffer from insomnia due to stress.

Feeling that there is nothing that you can do about the stress that you are facing in your life is perfectly normal. Our bills are going to continue coming, we are never going to feel as if there are enough hours in the day to get all of the things done that we need to get done, our families and our jobs are going to continue to demand our attention, and our to-do lists are going to continue to get longer.

Believe it or not, you do have some control in these situations. Simply realizing that you are in control of your own life is going to help you to begin managing your stress so that you can start sleeping at night.

Managing your stress is all about taking control of your life through the lifestyle that you live, taking control of your thoughts as well as your emotions, and learning how to deal with problems better.

It does not matter how much you have to deal with in your life or how much stress you have, there are things that you can do in order to regain control of your life and reduce the stress that you have to deal with on a regular basis.

It is very important for us to learn how to manage our stress because when we live with constant high levels of stress, we are putting our physical and mental health at risk. Too much stress reduces our ability to function in day to day life, think clearly, or just enjoy life in general.

When we learn how to manage our stress though, we break the hold that it has on our lives. This allows us to not only be healthier but happier as well as more productive. Our goal should be to learn how to balance our lives. We have to find time for our work, to focus on our relationships, to take care of all of our responsibilities, and to relax as well as have fun. We also have to learn how to deal with the pressure that we are going to face that is not planned for and face the challenges that show up in our lives.

When it comes to stress management there is not one single thing that I can tell you to do that is going to work for every person. This is because the stress that we all face is very different in all of our lives. What may cause one person stress may not cause another to. While one person may be stressed in one area of their lives another person may be dealing with stress in another area of their lives.

This means that while some of these tips may work for you some of them may not. Don't be afraid to try them all and figure out what works best for you in your situation.

1. Start by identifying the source of the stress that you are dealing with in your life. If you are dealing with stress in just one area of your life you will want to identify that area. For example, if you have recently changed jobs, if you are moving, if you are having problems in your relationship, or if you are having financial issues.

   Understanding where the stress is coming from is very important if you want to learn how to manage it.

   It is very easy to overlook the things that are causing us stress in our lives. We tend to forget that we are people too and expect so much out of ourselves that we may not realize where the stress is coming from. If this is the case, take a look at what is going on in the different areas of your life. For example, are you not cleaning your house as you should? Perhaps you are not meeting your deadlines? Is there one area of your life that you are always procrastinating in?

   If you find that you are regularly struggling in one area of your life this could be the area that is causing you stress. On the other hand, you may be struggling in one area because another area is demanding so much of your time. Take an honest look at your life and determine where the stress is coming from.

2. Decide what you can take control of. While there are things that you cannot control, for example, how your in-laws

behave or the way that your boss acts at work, there are things that you can take control of. You can control how you will react to certain situations, how productive you are going to be, how you are going to spend your time and how you will spend your money.

It is important for you to be able to decipher what you can control and what you cannot control. The worst thing that you can do for your stress is to try and take control over things that you have no control over. If you try to do this, you are going to fail and that is only going to cause you to feel more stress.

Once you have determined what is causing you stress, you need to focus on the things in those specific areas that you can control. This is the best way for you to determine what action you will need to take in order to reduce your stress. For example, if you are dealing with a lot of stress because of the number of responsibilities that you have at home, try talking to your partner about it and handing some of the responsibility over to them.

Stress can make us feel as if our power in our lives has been taken away. When we focus on the things that we can change, we are taking some of that power back.

3. Do the things you love. Find something that you love to do and spend time doing it. It is easy to allow one area of our lives that we are dealing with a lot of stress to take over the

rest of our lives. However, taking the time to do something we love will help us manage those other areas that are causing us stress. Doing something that you love is going to allow you to take your mind off of the things that are stressing you out which will result in your body being able to relax. This will lead to much better sleep.

4. Learn how to manage your time. One of the biggest reasons that people find themselves over-stressed is because they do not feel as if they have enough time to get everything done that needs to be done. They have a to-do list that is a mile long, but it seems that there are not enough hours in the day to even work on it.

Why is it that some people seem to be able to do everything? They excel at their jobs, have a side gig, are great parents and partners, their house is always clean, their bills are always paid, and they always look great? It seems that there are people out there who have more time than other people do. The truth is that we all have the same 24 hours in each day. It is up to us what we do with them. There are plenty of people out there who are sleeping 7 to 8 hours a night and still getting everything done that they need to get done while having time for their family, friends and fun.

Take some time and write down everything that you do in one day. Don't write down things that you want to do or that you do not normally do. Be honest with yourself and only write down what you actually do. Next to each task, write down the number of hours that it takes you to do them.

On another sheet of paper, write down each hour of the day, leaving some space between them, starting with the time that you get up and ending with the time that you go to bed. Now write in all of the tasks that you do at the time that you do them, blocking out the amount of time that it takes to do them. For example, if you work from 8 a.m. to 4 p.m. every day, block that time out just for work.

How much time is left where there is nothing written? Most people will find that they have a lot of time left when they thought they had none at all. The reason that this happens is that we end up wasting a lot of our time.

Have you ever considered how many hours each week you actually sit scrolling through social media on your phone? Or how many hours you sit playing games on your devices? What about the number of hours each week that you spend watching television? All of this time adds up. Even if it is just 30 minutes per day per activity that is still 90 minutes, for just these three activities. How many other unproductive activities are you taking part in each day?

Think about the other things that you could be doing instead of wasting your time. You could be spending time with your kids at the park, going to the gym, hanging out with your friends, or even working on that project that you wanted to finish.

When we take control of our time, we often find that we have time to spend doing the things that we love and that is going to help reduce the stress in the other areas of our lives. When we spend time doing what we enjoy we are going to find that the thing that is causing us stress does not cross our minds. This gives our minds a break and allows them to rest which will lead to better sleep.

5. Prepare for the stress that you are going to face in your life by knowing how you are going to handle it. Deep breathing is a great way to destress when you are standing in the grocery store checkout line and the person in front of you seems to be taking 10 times longer than they should. However, there are times when deep breathing isn't the answer. Perhaps the answer is writing out the problem as well as all of the solutions. Or managing your time better. Knowing how you will manage difficult situations is going to help reduce the stress in your life and as we have already learned, this will lead to better sleep.

6. Decide what you are going to do, what can wait, and what someone else can do. I understand if you are one of those people that would rather do everything on their own because that is the only way that you will know for sure that it is done the right way. I am one of those people. One thing that I have learned is that you can't do everything on your own.

Sometimes you have to decide what you are going to do and let other people pick up the slack. You shouldn't feel as if everything is your responsibility.

If you are working 7 days a week, taking care of the house and kids when you come home, preparing all of the meals, paying all of the bills, and doing all of the grocery shopping when you are at home, your stress level is going to be so high that you are not going to be able to relax. Choose the things that you are going to do each day. If you don't have time to prepare all of the meals, delegate that task to someone else. Have someone do laundry while you shower at night or have someone do the dishes after dinner while you help the kids with their homework.

Not only is this going to help you get a little more, free time but it is going to take all of the stress off of your shoulders.

No one should have to carry the weight of the world on their shoulders and that includes you. Look for things in your life that are causing you more stress than they are worth. Do your kids really need to do 4 extracurricular activities? Do you really need to volunteer 3 times a week? What can you do in order to reduce the number of things on your plate?

Often times we find that we are the biggest cause of our own stress. We think that we can take on so much more than we can handle. We have to remember that we are only human. If you are doing more than you would expect from anyone else perhaps it is too much. It might be time to start cutting back.

7. Are you opening yourself up to more stress? When we don't take the time to take care of ourselves, we are opening ourselves up to more stress. Of course, this is going to lead to less sleep which will circle around again leading to more stress. Are you getting enough exercise or are you sitting on the couch all of the time? Are you skipping meals in hopes of using that time to get things done around the house? Do you have more projects going than you can handle? Are you too stubborn to ask for help?

   All of these are going to open us up to more stress in our lives which is going to affect our health. Too much stress can cause many different physical health problems as well as mental health problems. It can cause us to suffer from insomnia. If you are leaving yourself open to more stress you have to start taking action right now in order to stop.

8. Set boundaries. If you are the type of person that has a hard time telling people no, the chances are that you are under a huge amount of stress. I used to be that person but let me tell you what I learned. Over the years I learned that as long as you keep giving people are going to keep taking. If you keep allowing them to demand your time, they are going to keep demanding of your time.

At some point, you have to put your foot down and say, "Enough is enough." You have to start putting yourself first and stop taking on everything that everyone else wants you to do.

One thing that I have learned about being productive and living a happy life is that I have to focus on what is going to make me happy in my life. I cannot focus on what is going to make everyone else in the world happy. Of course, my family's happiness goes along with my own because if they are not happy, I could not be happy. As for everyone else, their happiness is their own responsibility.

I know that this may sound cold but at some point, we have to stop trying to please everyone and decide that we are important enough to be happy as well. Saying no is going to take a lot of stress off of you. It is going to give you the time that you want to spend with your family or to go do all of the fun things that you want to do.

You are not being mean by saying no and you are not letting someone down. You are taking a stand for yourself and saying that you are important too. Trust me someone else will always be there to say yes so don't feel like no one is going to be there to fill the void.

9. We have to understand that caring and worrying are two different things. Worrying is going to cause stress in your

life. When you spend time worrying about something it is because you want to have control over the situation.

"I worry about what you do when you are out with your friends," = "I want to control what you do when you are out with your friends."

See how that works. Caring on the other hand means that we just want what is in the best interest of something or someone.

"I care about you." = "I want what is best for you."

Worrying does not involve any action. It simply means that you are causing yourself stress over something that you do not have control of. Caring on the other hand means that you do take action.

If you worry about your health, the chances are that it is all you do, worry that something will go wrong. If you care about your health, you are going to take action to make sure that your body is healthy.

There really is no point in worrying. Sitting around and mentally fussing over something that you have no control over is simply pointless. I am sure that there are much better things that you would like to do with your time.

If you want to improve your sleep, stop spending time in bed focusing on something that you have no control over.

Instead, accept that you have no control over the situation and move on to things that you can actually take action on.

10. Accept your mistakes and stop trying to be perfect. Perfectionism… If you suffer from it, you understand just how hard it can make your life. If you can't give something your all you don't see any point in trying. If you can't do something perfectly you don't want to do it. Perfection is something that we can strive for and we should strive for, but it is also something that we have to understand we will never reach.

Trying to do everything perfectly is going to reduce the amount of success that you have. It is going to cause more stress in your life, and it is going to make you feel as if you are never good enough.

You have to accept that good enough is good enough. Things are rarely going to work out perfectly in life. When they do that is great but don't get discouraged because they don't. Accept that you did well and that is all anyone could ask for.

As a perfectionist, you are going to have to start looking at yourself as a person. You are a human just like everyone else. You don't expect everyone else to do things perfectly so why would you expect that of yourself. We have to treat ourselves like we would a friend because we are the best friend that we will ever have.

Stop comparing yourself to other people. This world that we live in is filled with filters and edits. You only see the parts of people's lives that they want you to see. You only see the best pictures of them when their makeup is perfect. Or when they choose the right filter.

You cannot compare yourself to a filtered version of someone else and you cannot compare your life to a filtered version of someone else's life. Instead, compare you to you.

How far have you come in the past year? What changes have you made in your life? What improvements do you see in your own life or relationships? When we stop comparing ourselves to the filtered versions of everyone else, we see that we don't have to be perfect.

Focus on doing what you think is right. Chances are if you think you are doing the right thing, you will be doing the right thing. It does not matter if everyone else says that it is okay to do something and you feel that it is not, do what you feel is best for you. When you start putting yourself first and doing what feels right to you, you will no longer feel the need to be perfect at everything that you do.

Finally, create an environment that allows you to simply be a person. Don't surround yourself with a bunch of perfectionists because perfectionism can be contagious. If you spend all of your time with people who feel the need to be perfect, you are going to feel the need to be perfect as well.

This does not mean that you should spend all of your time with unmotivated lazy people either. Instead, try to meet some people who fall right in the middle. Balanced. That is what you are aiming for.

You want to continue to stay motivated but not to the point of perfection.

What you are going to see as you overcome your perfectionism is that your stress levels are reduced dramatically. You are going to see more success than you have ever seen before and you are going to start enjoying your life.

Remember that you don't have to have it all in life to be happy. It is possible for every single person on this planet to be happy with what they have no matter how little or how much it is because what we have is not what makes us happy. Who we are and the things that we do is what affects our happiness.

11. Stay away from people who cause you stress. We all have those people in our lives, just walking into a room with them seems to cause our stress levels to rise. They are the people who feel the need to complain about everything that is going on in their lives. They are constantly focused on the negative. Or their behavior is so outrageous that we simply cannot stand to be in the same room with them for more than 5 minutes.

Did you know that you have control over the people that you are around? Of course, if the people who cause you stress are at work you don't have much control over it, however that does not mean that you can't stay away from them. Simply avoid them in a polite way. Don't sit with them in the break room, don't go out to lunch with them, if they come up to talk to you, politely tell them that you have to send an email or answer a text and then walk away. You decide who is in your life.

12. Learn how to express your feelings. This is very hard for a lot of people. We bottle our emotions up when something is bothering us when we should be communicating our feelings. What happens is that we become so stressed that we are not able to manage in our day to day lives. Our emotions keep building up and just like a shaken soda bottle, the lid pops off and all of our emotions come pouring out, usually at the worst time.

If you notice that things are starting to bother you, instead of bottling your emotions up and letting them out all at once, talk to whoever is the cause of the situation. Learn how to communicate instead of building resentment towards those that are causing you stress. For example, if you are busy working on a project and your husband keeps coming into the room interrupting you, instead of getting angry and bottling up those emotions, simply tell him that you are working, you have to get the project done, and he can have your full attention when you are finished. Remind him that the more he interrupts you, the longer the project is going to take. Chances are, he will understand.

You don't have to bottle up your emotions in order to protect other people's feelings. You are allowed to feel however you feel even if it upsets someone else.

It does not matter what you do, you are always going to have stressors in your life. You will always have things or people in your life that are going to cause you stress. In order to ensure that this stress does not affect your health or your sleep, you will have to learn how to manage it. When we learn how to manage our stress, we will find that it affects our lives less and we are not focused on it all of the time.

If you live a very stressful life and have not been managing your stress properly you may find that just by using the tips above, you will start sleeping better at night. Of course, managing your stress should be part of the bigger picture though. You cannot focus on just one area of your life and hope that by making a few changes your insomnia is going to go away.

You have to realize that your entire life is affecting your sleep which is why we are addressing each area in this book. Making small changes in each area will be what leads you to a better night's sleep.

Chapter 8

Creating the
Environment for Sleep

❀ ❀ ❀ ❀ ❀ ❀ ❀ ❀ ❀ ❀ ❀ ❀ ❀ ❀ ❀

The way that your bedroom is set up may not seem like a very big deal. Most people do not take their sleep environment into consideration when they are suffering from insomnia. Improving your sleep environment may be the best way for you to reduce your insomnia quickly allowing you to get the rest that you need. Your sleep environment is the area where you want to be sleeping. Most of the time your sleep environment is your bedroom.

You can learn a lot about someone from looking at their bedroom. You may find that while they do wash their laundry on a regular basis it is not getting put away. Or that they went on a business trip, camping is something that they enjoy, or that they go through six outfits each morning before they find the right one.

No two bedrooms are the same. Of course, most of them will contain the same types of furniture but each bedroom is unique to the person sleeping in them. This means that not everyone is going to agree on what their sleep environment should be like. When two people are sharing the same sleep environment it can be difficult to set up the sleep environment in a way that allows both partners to rest. Often times this leads to problems within the relationship.

Clutter In Your Sleep Environment

Have you ever gone to bed at night feeling poorly about the condition of your bedroom? Many people find that the tidiness, or untidiness of their bedrooms affect their sleep.

A messy bedroom often means a messy life. Usually those that have a messy bedroom have things that they have not completed that they know they need to get done, yet, instead of finishing those projects or tasks, they end up piled up in the bedroom. This leads to poor sleep.

We spend about a third of our lives in bed which means that we spend more time in our bedrooms than we do in any other room in our houses. Of all of the rooms in the house that should be clutter-free, the bedroom is the most important. Clutter can cause a person to feel anxious which will prevent them from getting the sleep that they need.

A cluttered bedroom is uncomfortable and can even lead to depression. Studies have actually shown that having a messy bedroom can affect your entire day. People with messy bedrooms are not as productive as those that have clean bedrooms. They are less able to focus on the tasks that they need to get done and their relationship with their partner suffers due to the mess.

The very first thing that you need to do in order to create a sleep environment that promotes sleep is to clean. Your bedroom should be one of the cleanest rooms in your home. Make sure that it is free from clutter. Take all of those sports equipment, camping gear, or stuff for your other hobbies and find a new place to store them.

Do not pile laundry up in your room. It does not matter if the laundry has been washed or if it is still dirty, it does not belong in your room. Waking up and seeing all of those clothes will only cause you stress first thing in the morning. Keep all of your paperwork out of your bedroom. Find a place in your home where you will file your paperwork and complete any paperwork that needs to be completed.

Remove anything from your room that has to do with your job. You do not need your briefcase in your room, nor do you need your laptop.

Cleaning your room and keeping it clean is very important to your sleep. Make sure that you are changing your sheets once per week and washing all of your blankets on a regular basis. Make your bed every day. While making your bed each morning before you do anything else does promote productivity, if you can't bring yourself to do this, just make sure that your bed is made before you get into it at night. It is going to make you sleep better and feel better about the space that you are in.

Too Much Noise

When it comes to noise in the bedroom the quieter the better. Sleeping is much easier to do when you are in a quiet environment. This is why many people have found that they sleep better when they go out camping in the woods. There is no noise to distract us from sleep or to keep us up at night.

We cannot stop our bodies from responding to noises when we are trying to sleep. You see, if we were sleeping in a cave, we would need our bodies to respond to sounds in order to ensure our own safety. Even though we no longer sleep in caves our bodies still respond the same way to noises when we are asleep. This means that if the neighbor has their music turned all the way up until 3AM our bodies are not going to let us go to sleep. While we can hear noises while we are sleeping and not fully wake up, we are pulled out of deep sleep which affects how much rest we are getting.

If you cannot control the amount of noise in your sleep environment, try finding a way to reduce it as much as possible. You can use a fan or a white noise machine to help reduce the amount of outside noise that you hear. Or you can use earplugs to block out all of the noise. If you have children, I do not suggest wearing earplugs. As a parent you probably understand why but it is important for you to be able to hear those little calls for you in the middle of the night.

Some people suggest turning your television on at a low volume in order to reduce outside noises, but I do not suggest this at all. Adding more noise is not going to help you sleep better but instead it is going to cause it to be harder for you to fall asleep at night and it can cause you to wake up often during the night.

It's Hot In Here

The majority of people are going to find that they sleep better in a cooler room. While you may end up buried under 10 blankets there is something about the cool air that helps some people sleep better.

On the other hand, there are those who seem to be freezing all of the time and find it much easier to doze off in a warm room. If you are sharing a bed with someone who prefers it to be cool and you need it to be warm, it can be hard for you to find the perfect temperature for your sleep environment.

You don't want to wake up in the middle of the night shivering and you don't want to wake up so hot that you cannot breathe. Why? Because waking up in the middle of the night is a problem when you are not getting enough sleep.

In order to find the best temperature for sleep, think about how the temperature changes outside. It is cooler at night than it is during the day. Our bodies work in the same way. Our internal temperature will drop a bit during the night in order to preserve energy. This means that you are going to benefit from having a cooler sleep environment.

Play around with the temperature in your bedroom. Sleep in the coolest temperature that you can. This is going to help you get more sleep and it is going to help you sleep better. Of course, if you need 10 blankets piled on top of you pile them on.

Most people do not like to wake up to a cold house, especially in the wintertime. Instead of waking up to a cold house you can use a programmable thermostat to start increasing the temperature in your home just before you have to get out of bed. This way, you will not be shivering as you make your way through the house each morning.

Light

The amount of light that is in our sleep environment is going to play a huge role in how well we are sleeping. Your body is going to rest better when you are sleeping in the dark. Some people like to have some sort of nightlight, especially if they find that they are getting up during the night to go to the bathroom. This is okay but it would be best if the light is outside of the bedroom.

Our bodies naturally want to sleep when it is dark outside. This can make it hard for people that are working overnights. Most people who work overnights will try to make their room as dark as possible when they are sleeping because they understand that light is what keeps them awake. Even the light from your electronics can affect you the same way that light from the sun would, causing your body to believe that it is time for you to stay awake.

This is why it is so important for you to remove all electronics from your bedroom. It is okay for you to charge your phone on your bedside table if you use it as an alarm, however, the best option would be to actually invest in an alarm clock and charge your phone overnight in another room so that you are not tempted to pick it up and expose yourself to the blue light.

Remove the television from your bedroom as well. This can be hard for a lot of people and I completely understand why. Most of us do not have enough time in our days to sit down and watch television. The only time that we have to catch up on our favorite television shows is when we are lying in bed at night. Even if this means just catching a few minutes before we doze off, we feel like this is our time to relax.

Unless you are completely exhausted and pushing your body to its limits, when you are exposed to the blue light from the television you are going to have a hard time falling asleep. We talked in an earlier chapter about how the blue light from electronics affects sleep in the same way that the sunlight does. Television does the same thing. Taking the television as well as all other electronic devices out of the bedroom will help you to get a better night's sleep. Make sure that you are turning all of your screens off at least one hour before you go to bed in order to make sure you are getting the best sleep possible.

Your Bed

Different people sleep in different ways. Each culture has its own bedding preferences. Each of them will provide you with benefits. The truth is that there is no right or wrong way for a person to sleep. It all depends upon your personal preferences and what is most comfortable for you.

One thing that you have to think about when it comes to the way that you are sleeping is the bed that you are sleeping on. Is your mattress soft enough that it is not causing you pain when you are trying to sleep? Is it firm enough to support your back? Is your mattress the right size? Do you have enough space on your mattress to sleep comfortably without feeling crowded or having any part of your body hanging off of the bed?

When you are sleeping your comfort is very important. If you are sleeping on a mattress that is not comfortable for you, this could affect your sleep. The situation can become complicated if you are sharing your bed with a partner because what is comfortable to them may not be comfortable for you.

If you find that the bed that you are sleeping on is causing you sleep problems, a new mattress may be in order. You don't have to go out and buy the most expensive bed in the market. You may first want to try a mattress topper if the bed is too hard for you to sleep on.

You may be most comfortable sleeping with just a sheet on you or you may find that having lots of thick blankets helps you to get the most sleep. Don't feel as if you have to sleep a certain way because that is what you were always told. Instead, experiment with the way that you sleep and find what works best for you.

The Bedroom Is For Sleeping

Many people find that they have turned their bedrooms into multipurpose rooms. We hide away in our bedrooms in order to get extra work done in the evening, we spend time reading books in our bedrooms, watching television, budgeting, meal planning, and the list goes on.

The bedroom needs to be a place where you go to rest. It should not be a place where you do things that cause you stress or that stimulate you. Bedrooms should be used specifically for sex and sleep, nothing else. You do not need to be doing your work in your bedroom. Find another area of the house even if it means that you are working at the kitchen table. You do not need to be playing games or watching television when you are in your bedroom. Do not bring the stresses of your everyday life into your bedroom. Instead, make your bedroom an area that is free from all of those stressors, a place where you can go to relax. This is going to make it much easier for you to fall asleep and stay asleep.

Smells and Sleep

The different scents that we smell throughout the day affect us much more than we think. Did you know that the scents that are in your bedroom can affect your sleep? Studies have shown that the scents in our environment can stimulate us, causing us to be more alert or they can calm us and help us relax. They can also cause us stress if we are not careful. This is why so many people have turned to aromatherapy in order to treat many different issues such as stress, insomnia, and chronic fatigue.

The first thing that you need to do in your bedroom after you have cleaned it is to think about the scents that you will be smelling as you are going to bed at night. You do not want to smell unpleasant scents all night long. For example, if you have a dog in the home, you do not want to smell the scent of dog all night as you are trying to sleep. We love our dogs and they are part of our family, but they smell. No one wants to smell unpleasant scents all night long.

In order to keep unpleasant smells out of your bedroom, you need to first make sure that you are keeping it clean. A clean environment is not going to smell. If you have pets or a partner who tends to have smelly shoes, you can use plugin air fresheners, fabric refreshers, diffusers, candles, or incents to make your sleep area smell better.

The smell of the room is not the only important thing when it comes to air. It is important to make sure that the air quality is good as well. If it is possible you should open your windows on occasion for a little while in order to allow fresh air into your home, making sure that you open your bedroom windows. If you are unable to open your windows don't worry. You can use an air purifier in order to keep the air clean.

The air purifier is going to help to remove pet dander, dust, and smoke from the room. You may also want to place a few plants in your room as well in order to improve the quality of the air.

The amount of humidity that is in the air is going to affect how your breathing which will affect how you sleep as well. If your room is too dry, you may want to run a humidifier on the other hand if there is too much humidity in the air, you may consider running a dehumidifier.

Taking the time to ensure that your sleep environment is supporting sleep is going to help you to reduce insomnia that you are suffering from and allow you to fall asleep faster and stay asleep longer. Making these small changes to your bedroom will promote better sleeping and could end your suffering completely, at the very least it will improve your sleep.

When you add in a sleep environment that supports sleep to all of the other changes that you are making in order to improve your sleep you are going to quickly find yourself falling asleep faster and staying asleep longer.

Chapter 9

Exercise and Sleep

"I just can't seem to fall asleep at night."
"How much exercise are you getting?"
"Exercise..."

Studies have shown that exercise will help you get better sleep at night. Exercise has so many benefits. It improves our overall health, provides us with extra energy, helps to reduce stress in our lives, and can improve the quality of sleep that we are getting.

Yet, today so many people don't exercise. Why? If you ask people why they do not exercise, many of them will tell you that they are too tired to exercise, they don't have enough time, they don't enjoy exercising, they are afraid to exercise because of some health issue, or that the weather stops them from exercising.

If you ask a hundred different people why they do not exercise, they can all come up with a hundred different reasons. The truth is that exercise simply is not important to them.

Our bodies were meant to move but today we live in a sedentary world. Much of our work is done behind a screen. We sit for the majority of our day while we complete our work. We go home and we end up sitting some more. We no longer take walks after dinner with the family because in most areas it just is not safe enough to do this or because we don't have enough time.

We are all so busy and we tell ourselves that there is not enough time to exercise. Remember when I had you write down all of the things that you had to do in one day and then write it all down on an hourly schedule? The chances are that you found yourself with a lot more free time than you thought you had. What are you going to do with that free time now that you know you have it available to you?

What you may have found while you were creating that schedule is that you are wasting a lot of your time. Perhaps spending a little too much time on social media when you should be working therefore causing yourself to have to work into the late hours of the night in order to meet deadlines. You may have found that you are spending far too much time sitting in front of the television or playing games on your devices when you could be doing something more productive such as exercising.

Go back and take a look at that schedule. Can you fit 3 hours per week for exercise if it means that you are going to be sleeping better at night?

Some people are going to say that they have tried to start exercising and it never worked out for them. In order to see the benefits of exercise, you have to stick with it. You can't exercise for one week and then expect to reap the benefits for the rest of your life.

It is best to exercise 1 hour per day at least 3 times per week. If you can work up to exercising 1 hour per day every day of the week, you are going to find that your sleep improves drastically.

Think about it like this…

Your body is made to move. Yet we sit at a desk all day long or we sit in front of the television. The only time that we move is to go from one seat to the next. We are eating lots of food that is providing our body with lots of energy, but this energy is not burned off as we move from one seat to the next.

Instead, this energy keeps building up as we go throughout our day. When we get home from work at night, we go again from one seat to the next, usually the couch. Then we go from the couch to the kitchen table and often right back to the couch.

How can you expect your body to be tired from doing almost nothing all day long? Sure, you were awake, and you were using your mind but not your body. Then you go to bed at night and your body does not feel tired. It does not feel the need to go to sleep because you have yet to burn off all of that energy that it has provided you with.

I see it all of the time. People come to me complaining that they are not able to sleep at night but when I ask them about exercise, they tell me that they are not exercising. Or they feel like they are getting enough physical exercise when in reality they are getting very little.

Don't get me wrong, moving your body all day long is important. While the things that you do each day do take a little energy, such as cleaning the house or running into the grocery store, they are not going to burn off enough energy for your body to be tired. You have to exercise enough each day for your body to want to rest if you want to sleep well.

Sleep is going to improve dramatically when you start exercising. You will see that your sleep is more restorative. This is because you are going to be spending more time in deep sleep. Deep sleep is the sleep stage that allows your body to recover. It helps to reduce stress, improve heart health and the immune system.

On top of the quality of your sleep improving you are going to see that you are sleeping longer while waking up less often during the night. When you exercise you are burning energy which is going to ensure that your body is ready to rest at the end of the day which means that your body will naturally sleep longer.

Exercise is also going to help you to reduce the amount of anxiety and stress that you are dealing with on a day to day basis. We talked earlier about how stress can cause sleep problems. What we did not cover was how exercise could help reduce that stress. Exercising for just 5 minutes causes anxiety and stress to begin lowering. It helps to clear the mind and helps you to break free from the fight or flight state.

There is scientific proof that shows exercise to be a natural remedy for insomnia. Aerobic exercise is the best type of exercise that a person with insomnia can do. Studies have shown though that instead of the benefits of exercise starting immediately, it takes time for them to build up. This means that you have to stick with exercising while you are suffering from insomnia, as well as continue exercising even after you start to see benefits.

How To Start Exercising

Exercising is one of the best things that a person can do for themselves, their health, and their quality of sleep. When you first start exercising it is going to take a little bit of time for you to start to see the benefits, but before long you are going to feel healthier and you are going to be sleeping better as well as longer.

It is going to take some determination and dedication for you to stick to a workout plan but if you really want to start sleeping as I am sure that you do, I promise you that it is going to be worth it.

You may be completely on board with exercising but don't know where to start. Perhaps you have never tried starting an exercise routine before and find it a little overwhelming. There is nothing wrong with that. I am going to give you the tools that you need so that you can start exercising, stick to your routine, and start sleeping better in no time.

1. See A Doctor- Before you can start exercising you need to see a doctor. Your doctor is going to be able to determine due to any health conditions that you suffer from, what

exercises you can and cannot participate in. If you already have health problems, it is very important for you to talk to your doctor before you begin any exercise program. Your doctor is also going to be able to tell if you are at risk of injury while you are exercising. They will provide you with this information and ensure that you know which exercises are safe for you.

This is going to allow you to create a workout that will work for you without pushing you beyond your limitations.

2. Set Goals- We accomplish nothing in our lives without first setting a goal. The main goal that you should have is to exercise for 1 hour per day. That is what you are working towards. This is not where you are going to start out.

Once you have that goal you are going to want to break it down into much smaller goals that you are going to be able to reach. For example, you may decide that you can start by working out for 15 minutes a day 3 times each week. That is a great place to start. As this becomes easier for you, you can add more time and then eventually add more days until you reach your goal of working out an hour per day.

Starting out small is going to increase your chances of succeeding. So many people want to jump right in to exercising for an hour each day, but they do not realize that they are setting themselves up for failure.

In the beginning exercise is new. It is not something that you have made a habit out of and it is not something that your muscles are used to. When you try to exercise for 1 hour per day right off the bat, you are going to find that your muscles are very sore. You are going to start making excuses not to exercise and before you know it, you are going to stop exercising all together.

I want you to benefit from exercise. I want you to be able to sleep better at night. That is why I want you to succeed in making exercise a habit. Start off small and work your way up.

3. Make it a habit- Doing exercise a habit is a key to your success. The longer that you exercise, the easier it is going to be for you to do. I am not talking just about physically. I am talking about convincing yourself to get up and go exercise.

Choose a specific time of the day to dedicate just to exercise. Do not schedule anything else during this time. For the next 30 days, I want you to focus on exercising at this time. Do not make excuses as to why you cannot exercise because that is what this time is dedicated to.

When you exercise at the same time every day, your body is going to get very used to going and exercising at that time. Before you know it, you will make exercise a habit and it will be as routine as brushing your teeth.

4. Choose an exercise that you enjoy and one that works for you. Perhaps you love to dance, or maybe walking on the treadmill while watching your favorite television show is going to work better for you, or perhaps you want to go walk in the park for an hour each morning as the sun comes up.

Find something that you really enjoy doing. When you enjoy the type of exercise that you are doing, you are more likely to stick with the exercise. You don't have to do the same thing every day either. Some days, when it is really cold or rainy outside, I will use my treadmill while I listen to podcasts. On other days I will go to the park and walk or go for a hike. Then there are days when all I want to do is play so I'll grab my jump rope and head outside with the kids.

You see, it doesn't really matter what you are doing, as long as you are getting exercise. In the beginning, when exercise is not part of your daily life, it is important for you to plan ahead. You will want to make sure that you know what exercise you are going to be doing in the time that you have set aside for exercise.

If later in the day, you are feeling energized enough to go jump rope or ride bikes, go for it. The more exercise you do, the better you are going to sleep.

Make sure that you are staying hydrated. Not only is this going to affect your health and your recovery time from the exercising that you are doing but it is going to affect your sleep as well. If you really want to sleep well, you have to take care of your body. That includes making sure that you are getting enough to drink each day.

When you first start exercising it can be easy to forget to warm up. If you are walking as your form of exercise, you will want to walk at a normal pace for about five minutes. Then you will take the time to stretch.

After you have finished exercising you will also need to take the time to cool down. This means that you will go back to walking at a normal pace for no less than 5 minutes and then you will stretch once again.

This is going to help prevent injury as you are exercising as well as allowing your body to return to its normal state.

You also need to make sure that you are listening to your body when you start working out. If you are not used to exercising every day, you need to pay attention to what your body is telling you. If your muscles become sore, you need to accept that and allow them a day to recover before exercising again. If you feel pain when you are exercising you need to be able to recognize what has caused that pain in order to prevent injury.

Exercise is meant to help you become healthier and to sleep better. It is not meant to cause you pain or injury.

Motivation

Staying motivated is vital if you want to stick to any exercise routine. If you are not motivated you will start putting exercise off, you may start coming up with excuses as to why you cannot exercise, or you will just quit exercising altogether.

If you find that you are having a hard time staying motived there are a few things that you can do.

- Make your goals more manageable. It is so easy for us to set unattainable goals when we start exercising. We are pumped, so motivated to start exercising but when we try to reach the enormous goals our motivation begins to dwindle quickly. Instead of trying to become insanely fit overnight, set smaller goals. Instead of trying to exercise for an hour a day, try exercising for 30 minutes or 15 if 30 is too much. Set more achievable reasonable goals for yourself in order to keep yourself motivated.

- Keep a journal. It is so easy for us to allow our progress to go unnoticed. Before you start exercising write down how you are sleeping at night. Write down how you feel during the day. Write down how you feel overall. Each day continues to write in your journal. At the end of one month, go back and look at how you felt on day one. Notice how much of a difference the exercise is making when it comes not only to your health but to the way that you are sleeping at night. Seeing how much your sleep has improved it going to help you feel motivated to continue to exercise even when you don't feel like it. You are going to be able to remind yourself how much better you are sleeping and how much exercise is helping you.

- Stop feeling guilty. Look, life happens and there are going to be times when you are just not going to be able to exercise the way that you want to. Just because you miss a day does not mean that you have to give up completely

- Stop comparing yourself to other people. It does not matter how much another person exercises each day. It does not matter how exercise is affecting their life. It does not matter what anyone else does or what is going on in their lives. The only thing that matters is what you are doing. It only matters that you are exercising in order to improve your health and the quality of your sleep. Be gentle with yourself and stop expecting of yourself what you think everyone else is doing.

- Have fun! Exercise can be torturous if you are doing things that you do not enjoy. Exercise should be fun. Do the things that you enjoy the most in order to ensure that you are getting the most out of your exercise and that you are staying motivated to keep exercising. You don't have to go to the gym to exercise if that is not something that you enjoy. You can dance in your living room or go hiking. The exercises that you are doing should feel like a break from all of the other demands that are on you and your life.

- Just get started. Tell yourself that you are going to exercise for just 10 minutes. Once those 10 minutes are over if you want to continue, keep going for another 5 minutes. You can continue to do this for up to 30 minutes if you are just starting out but do not go for more than one hour. Usually once you get started you will find that you are enjoying the activity and will want to continue doing it. The hardest part of doing anything is getting started. So, if you can just force yourself to get started, you will find the motivation to keep going.

- Make exercise convenient for you. If you don't want to drive across town to the park in order to exercise, hop on the treadmill. If you don't want to go out in the cold in order to exercise, grab a DVD and exercise along with it. Find things that you can fit into your day, even if it is just 30 minutes. If you have to, get up a little earlier in the morning in order to fit exercise in.

- Don't worry about the past. Who cares if you have never been the most athletic person that you know? Who cares if no one picked you to be on their teams for high school? That is all in the past. Be present. Focus on what you can do today. You don't have to be super athletic for your sleep to benefit from your exercise.

- Give yourself a reward. Go out and buy yourself a new outfit or go get a massage. Do something that you enjoy. You do not want to go out and eat something that is unhealthy though. Remember, while exercise is going to help improve your sleep it will also help to improve your overall health which is going to affect your sleep as well. Do not reward yourself with something that is going to undo the work that you have done.

Exercise helps us in many ways. It can help us to lose weight, become more productive, manage stress, and sleep better every night. When we suffer from insomnia it may be due to not getting enough exercise. Just one hour of exercise three times a week can help improve the quality of sleep that you are getting as well as help you stay asleep longer each night, which will benefit every area of your life.

It can be hard to stick to an exercise routine but reminding yourself of the benefits can help you to stay motivated to continue exercising even when you don't feel like it.

Chapter 10

Natural Remedies for Insomnia

Insomnia is a sleep disorder that many people suffer from every year. People find themselves struggling to fall asleep every night no matter how tired they may think that they are. They find that they are waking up all night long even though all they want to do is sleep. Insomnia can last for a few days or it can last for weeks or even months.

When a person suffers from insomnia every area of their life is affected. They are unable to focus on any task, their performance at work is usually poor which can lead to them losing their jobs, they become irritable, they suffer from fatigue, headaches, and can even develop depression as well as many other health problems.

There is help though. Throughout this book we have talked about many of the things that can be affecting your sleep causing you to suffer from insomnia and how you can improve your sleep.

While making changes to your life is very important especially if you are suffering from chronic insomnia or if you have found yourself suffering from insomnia often, getting some relief right now is important as well.

Throughout this chapter I am going to give you natural remedies that you can try tonight to help you get the rest that you need so that you can start making changes in the other areas of your life in order to promote better sleep.

1. Melatonin is often the first thing that people turn to when they are not able to fall asleep at night. Melatonin is a natural hormone that your body makes. You can get melatonin supplements at your pharmacy. It is very important that you make sure that you are purchasing a quality supplement. So many times, people lose faith in supplements such as melatonin because they are purchasing low-quality supplements that do not contain melatonin. Talk to your doctor before taking anything and ask them how much you should be taking each night.

   You can take melatonin 1 hour before you want to go to bed. This is going to help your body prepare for sleep just as it would if your body was producing the melatonin itself. If you purchase a high-quality supplement, you should find that you start to feel drowsy within the hour and that you sleep well during the night. When you wake up in the morning you should feel refreshed and not groggy.

   If you find that the supplement that you are taking is not working well for you, try switching to a different supplement or talk to your pharmacist about the different brands. Remember just because it is more expensive does not mean that it is of higher quality. Don't purchase your supplements at big box stores or at the grocery store. Try to get them at the pharmacy. Even if your big box store or grocery store has a pharmacy in it, the quality of the supplements is not going to be the same.

2. Nutmeg will help you fall asleep quickly because it has sedative properties. Warm up a cup of milk before you go to bed and sprinkle just 1/8 of a teaspoon of nutmeg powder into the milk. Drink this before you go to bed. Warm milk is going to help induce sleep and the nutmeg is going to boost the effects of the warm milk causing you to drift off to dreamland in no time.

   If warm milk does not appeal to you, then grab a glass of your favorite juice or even water and add ¼ of a teaspoon of nutmeg to it and drink it before you go to bed at night.

3. Cumin oil or seeds will also help with insomnia. You can make cumin tea to help with insomnia by heating 1 teaspoon of seeds on the stove over a low temperature for no more than 5 seconds. Then you will add in 1 cup of water to the seeds and bring it to a boil. Turn the heat off and allow the tea to cool for about 5 minutes. Strain out the seeds and drink the tea before you go to bed.

If tea is not your thing, simply sprinkle a banana with 1 teaspoon of cumin powder and enjoy before going to bed. Bananas are great for treating insomnia and the cumin powder will have you drifting off to sleep before you can even worry about having insomnia.

4. If you find that you like warm milk but want to mix things up a little or don't like nutmeg, try adding a bit of saffron and cinnamon powder to the milk. You can also add in 1 teaspoon of honey to create a super-powered tonic that is going to have you drifting off to sleep in no time.

5. Bananas are not only good for you, but they contain tryptophan as well. Simply eating a banana before going to bed can help to regulate your sleep. However, if you need a little more of a boost, place the banana in a pot of boiling water. Boil for 5 minutes and then remove the banana. Eat the inside of the banana drizzled with a bit of honey and drink the water that it was boiled in. In just 30 minutes you will find your eyelids getting heavy.

6. Cherry juice will help you sleep deeply every night. Drinking just one cup of cherry juice before you go to bed is going to help increase the amount of serotonin and melatonin that your body produces. These will cause your body temperature to lower as well as cause you to become drowsy which will lead to you falling asleep. Studies have shown that the majority of patients, no matter what the sleep disorder they were suffering from was, fell asleep in no

more than 90 minutes after drinking just one cup of cherry juice.

7. Most of us know how chamomile affects our sleep. We know that when we are stressed out, we can drink a cup of chamomile tea to help us relax, however, most of the time chamomile is overlooked as a treatment for insomnia.

    Drinking just one cup of chamomile tea one hour before bed can help you to relax as well as fall asleep.

    If you want to improve your mood or fight depression, you can add 2 tablespoons of dried lemon balm to your chamomile tea. This will help to lift your mood, promote relaxation, and help you feel calm before you go to bed.

8. Aromatherapy is a great way to help you get the sleep that you need. While aromatherapy is not going to cure your insomnia, because it is not treating the cause of insomnia, it can help you feel more relaxed and calmer as you get into bed each night, which can result in you falling asleep faster and staying asleep longer.

    There are many different ways that you can incorporate aromatherapy into your daily life in order to improve your quality of sleep. Placing a cotton ball on your bedside table that has a few drops of essential oils on it can help you fall asleep quickly. You don't have to invest a lot of money in order to use aromatherapy.

Placing just a few drops of chamomile oil or lavender oil on your cotton ball and placing it on your bedside table or close to your pillow at bedtime is going to help you to relax and drift off to sleep.

We have talked about how important scent is when it comes to getting the sleep that you need and how important it is for you to change your sheets and wash your bedding on a regular basis. What about in between washes? You can create your very own sleep-inducing bed spray to ensure that your bed smells great on those nights that the sheets are not washed.

You will need to get a 4-ounce spray bottle. The bottle should be dark in color and preferably glass. You will also need your favorite sleep-inducing or relaxing essential oil. I will cover the top essential oils for sleep in a moment. Place 40 drops of the essential oil into the 4-ounce spray bottle. Add in 3 ounces of distilled water. I also like to use distilled white vinegar because it is great at killing germs and viruses. If you do not like the smell of vinegar, don't worry water will work fine.

The essential oil will float to the top of the water every time that it is left to settle so you will need to shake it each time that you spray it or use a solubilizer in order to force the water and oil to mix. Simply spray your bedding each night before you go to bed.

You do not want to spray too much until you know how you are going to react to the essential oils. Spraying too much could lead to a headache or breathing problems. You just want to lightly mist your bedding.

Using essential oils in your bath is a great way to help you wind down before you go to bed at night. Essential oils will help you to relax and prepare for sleep. It is important to purchase high-quality essential oils that are safe for the skin.

You do not want to add the essential oils directly into the bath but instead, mix them with some Epsom salt or Dead Sea salt, then add the mixture to your bath. The salts are also going to help you to relax. Bath salts are great for muscle pains so if you are adding exercise to your routine in order to improve your sleep, your muscles will thank you for the bath salts.

It is important for you to avoid essential oils that stimulate the mind and body before you go to bed. Peppermint oil, lemon oil, orange oil, grapefruit oil, and any other oil that stimulates can make it harder for you to fall asleep. Save these oils for the daytime when you need an extra boost.

Just like most things in life, every person is going to react to different essential oils differently. While one may cause someone to fall asleep it may cause another person to stay awake. You will have to experiment a little with essential oils to find the ones that work best for you.

These are the most common essential oils to promote sleep:

Chamomile

Lavender

Sandalwood

Clary Sage

Mandarin

Bergamot

Fragonia

Ylang Ylang

Using essential oils is not meant to replace any medical advice from your doctor. It is meant to help boost your sleep as is all of the other techniques that you have found in this book. It is important to determine if you have an underlying condition that is causing you to suffer from insomnia by visiting your doctor.

9. St. John's Wort is another natural remedy for those who are suffering from insomnia. Many people who are dealing with depression take St. John's Wort in order to reduce the symptoms that they are suffering from. St. John's Wort is known for increasing the amount of serotonin in the brain. The more serotonin that you have in your body, the more melatonin you will produce. When you produce more melatonin, you will sleep better.

You can make a tea out of dried St. John's Wort flowers. Simply boil 8 ounces of water with 2 teaspoons of the dried flower. Strain the flower out of the tea and then add in honey or lemon if desired.

10. Catnip helps to relieve stress as well as anxiety, reduce pain, and induce sleep. Yes, you read that right, catnip. Now don't go raiding your cat's stash. You should focus on getting dried catnip or catnip that is meant for human consumption. If you are suffering from inflammation in the body which is causing it to be difficult for you to sleep, catnip might be the answer you have been looking for because it helps to reduce inflammation as well.

You can make some catnip tea to drink before you go to bed. Boil one cup of water and then add in 4 teaspoons of fresh catnip or 2 teaspoons dried. Allow the tea to sit for 10 minutes and then strain out the catnip. Drink before going to bed at night. You may add honey as well if desired.

Natural remedies are a great way to go if you find that you need that extra boost at night to help you fall asleep and to stay asleep. Even though these will help you to get the sleep that you need, it is still important for you to treat the cause of insomnia. For example, if it is stress that is causing you to suffer from insomnia you need to learn how to handle that stress. If you find that you have a medical condition that is making it hard for you to fall asleep you need to make sure that you are treating that condition and not just treating the symptoms.

Why Use Natural Remedies?

For hundreds of years people have sought out natural remedies for all sorts of ailments including insomnia. At least 50 percent of all adults have tried a natural remedy at some point in their life and if they have not tried one, they are likely to down the road.

Not all-natural remedies are the same nor are they effective. When you are using natural remedies, you need to make sure that you are using them alongside any treatment that your doctor has recommended. It is also important to understand that not all-natural remedies are safe.

I have spoken a few times about how important it is for you to ensure that the supplements that you take are of high quality. This is because some of the supplements that are on the market today, do not meet the safety requirements that have been set by the FDA. They are considered food by the FDA because they contain plants. This means that clinical trials are not required nor is the same testing that is done on other over the counter medication. The labels only have to follow the guidelines for food and not the same guidelines that over the counter medications have to follow.

This is why so many companies are getting away with selling supplements that do not actually contain any of what they claim it contains. Notice the *not evaluated by the FDA warning that is on the side of herbal supplements. This means that they can basically claim that these supplements will do anything and contain anything but in reality, they don't have to live up to that claim.

Once you take a quality supplement after taking one that is of poor quality, you are going to notice a huge difference.

Most of the time when a person tries a home remedy and finds that it is not working for them it is because of the low-quality ingredients that they are using. On top of all of this you have to talk to your doctor before you start taking any type of supplement or start using any type of home remedy to ensure that the ingredients will not interact with any medications that you are currently taking.

It is important to remember that natural remedies should not be a replacement for your medications. If your doctor has prescribed you medication, they have done so for a reason. Do not stop taking your medication just because you have started using a natural remedy. Instead, use the natural remedy on top of your medication. If at a later point your doctor decides that you no longer need to take the medication as long as you continue with the natural remedy that is something that the two of you can discuss.

Chapter 11

Over the Counter Medications and When to Talk To Your Doctor

You have followed all of the tips in this book, you have tried everything that you can think of to help with your insomnia yet you are still struggling to get a good night's rest, so you are starting to think about using an over the counter sleep aid.

Before you decide to use an over the counter medication in order to help you get the sleep that you desperately need, you have to understand that while they can be effective, they are not going to cure your insomnia. The majority of sleep aids that you can purchase are going to contain what is known as antihistamines. Antihistamines do help you to feel sleepy, however, our bodies build up a tolerance to them very quickly.

What many people find when they take an over the counter sleep aid is that even after you have slept all night you are still going to feel very tired the next day. It is also important to remember that not a lot of information is available when it comes to over the counter sleep aids so we don't really know how effective they are or what the side effects are going to be.

Options

Diphenhydramine often found in Aleve PM and Benadryl is an antihistamine that causes you to feel drowsy. You may find that this type of medication leads to drowsiness during the day, vision problems, dry mouth, and constipation. These are okay to take on occasion and work best if taken on a night where you do not have a lot going on the next day because they continue to make you drowsy into the next day.

Doxylamine succinate is another antihistamine and it can be found in Unisom Sleep Tabs. Because it is an antihistamine it has the same types of side effects as other antihistamines. You may end up suffering from drowsiness the next day as well as blurred vision, dry mouth, and constipation.

We talked briefly about melatonin in the last chapter. Melatonin occurs naturally in the body and its job is to regulate our sleep. It works great to help a person with insomnia fall asleep faster and stay asleep longer, however, it does not come without side effects. Some people report experiencing daytime drowsiness after taking melatonin or suffering from headaches the next day.

Talking To Your Doctor

Sleep disorders are broadly defined as any psychological or physical issue that affects your ability to sleep. Anyone can suffer from a sleep disorder at any time. If you find that:

You are having a hard time falling asleep or staying asleep on a regular basis,

You get tired during the day even when you have slept for 7 or more hours the previous night

You have a hard time completing normal daytime activities due to sleepiness.

You snore loudly or even stop breathing during the night.

You have a hard time staying awake when you are watching television or reading.

You struggle to maintain focus.

You are often told that you look as if you are very tired.

You have memory problems.

You feel unable to control your emotions.

You respond slowly.

You feel as if you have to take a nap just to get through the day.

You may be suffering from one or more sleep disorders.

If you feel that none of the techniques or remedies in this book have helped you with your sleep disorder, you will want to talk to your doctor. However, before you can talk to your doctor, there are a few things that you are going to need to do.

The first thing that you have to do is to keep a sleep diary. In this diary, you are going to want to write down the time that you are going to bed, about how long it is taking you to fall asleep, how long you are sleeping, how many times you wake up during the night, and how you feel the next morning.

A smartwatch would be very beneficial if you can afford one. It is going to tell you the exact minute that you fall asleep, how you are sleeping, as well as how often you are waking up at night.

In your journal, you will want to write down any issues that you were facing, or if you do not want to go into a lot of detail, simply write down if you are dealing with a lot of stress. Track what you were eating as well as the amount of caffeine or alcoholic drinks you have consumed. It is also important to make sure that you write down any medications that you have taken or any drugs that you are using.

You do have to remember that doctors often do not take sleep problems seriously and they may believe that you are just trying to get sleeping pills. This is why it is so important for you to go into your visit armed with the information listed above. Show your doctor that you take your sleep issues seriously and that you expect them to, as well.

Doctors also get very used to hearing people tell them that they are not getting enough sleep because it is a symptom of so many other health issues. Because of this, they may not fully hear what you are saying. This is when the sleep journal comes in handy.

Handing over the sleep journal will allow your doctor to take a few minutes to see exactly what it is that you are dealing with. The sleep journal is also going to help you to explain to your doctor what is going on. How many times have you thought that you were ready to see the doctor only to have your mind blank when they start asking you what is going on? The sleep journal is going to ensure that this does not happen to you.

You should also write down any of the techniques or remedies that you have tried from this book. Chances are if you go straight to the doctor without trying any of these techniques that is where they are going to start. They are not going to start off by giving you a prescription. Showing them that you did put in the work that you needed before coming to see them is a great way to show them how serious you are and it will ensure that you do not have to deal with unneeded additional steps before you get the help that you need.

The next thing that you will want to do is write down any questions that you have.

Having this list is going to ensure that you get the answers that you need. You do want to make sure that you keep the questions brief because your doctor has about 20 minutes to assess you and provide you with the answers that you need. Being prepared is going to ensure that those 20 minutes are spent wisely. Here are some sample questions:

1. What is causing me to suffer from insomnia?

There are many different reasons that a person can develop insomnia and it is important for you to know what is causing yours. If you do not know what is causing your insomnia it can make treatment very difficult.

2. Is it possible that insomnia is a symptom of something bigger?

Insomnia can be the symptom of an undiagnosed health problem. If insomnia is caused by another health problem, you want to make sure that the health problem is being addressed and not just the symptoms.

3. What will happen if my insomnia is untreated?

Insomnia is not life-threatening. When a person suffers from insomnia long term though it can cause many negative side effects as we discussed earlier in this book. Understanding this condition is very important because it is going to help you decide how you want it to be treated. You should also focus on the cause of insomnia. If the cause is not treated, then what is going to happen?

4. Is there anything that I can do in my own life, short of what I have already tried that could help improve my sleep? Your doctor may be able to provide you with more techniques that you can try in order to improve your insomnia. They may even find that it is one of your medications that is causing you to suffer from insomnia. By

simply making a change to your medication you may find that insomnia disappears.

5. Are there treatments available to me? Your options for treatment are going to depend on a number of things. Firstly, how your doctor feels about the treatments as well as how the treatments are going to affect you or interact with other medications that you are taking.

6. What are the side effects of this treatment? Whenever you start a new medication, it is important for you to understand what the side effects are. You need to know if the side effects are worse than the symptoms that you are already suffering from or if things are going to get better. Are the side effects worth taking the medication?

7. Is my insomnia going to go away? There is no magic pill that will cure your insomnia. Many people who suffer from insomnia find that they suffer from it for years. Finding the right treatment for your insomnia is going to take some time as well. If you have gone through every tip and remedy in this book than you already know that finding the best option for you will take time. While you are under the care of the doctor you have to make sure that you are communicating with them, letting them know what is working for you and what is not working. Ask your doctor how long it is going to take before you start seeing changes in your sleep patterns.

Follow whatever advice your doctor gives you. Their job is to treat you and focus on your health. They really do have your best interest in mind when they are providing you with different treatment options. When you do not do as your doctor has directed you are only slowing the treatment process down and hurting yourself. Even if you feel like what your doctor is telling you is not going to work, give it a shot anyway. They deal with a lot of people suffering from sleep disorders and they are going to start by providing you with the treatments that work the most often in their own experience.

Be assertive when you talk to your doctor. If you don't understand what they are saying let them know. If you feel as if they are not listening to you make sure that you speak up. This is your health that is on the line. Make sure that they know you are more than just another insurance payment.

The majority of sleep problems are going to be solved if you follow the information that you have learned in this book. If you follow all of the tips and tricks that you have learned about diet, exercise, your sleep environment, and so on, chances are you will find that your sleep is going to improve.

However, if you do everything that I have told you and you still find that your sleep has not improved, you will want to talk to your doctor.

Conclusion

The next step is to start working proactively to ensure that you are taking care of your own health in order to ensure that your body is functioning properly so that you can get the sleep that you need.

Most people don't want to admit to not putting their own health first, but we all know that it happens. We get busy, we grab quick unhealthy meals, we forget to exercise, we stay up late in order to get more work done, and our health seems to come second to everything else.

Think of insomnia as a warning. Your body is telling you something is not right, and you need to start paying attention to it. When you start taking care of you and your own body, you are going to find that it responds by taking care of you.

Most often, when a person suffers from insomnia, it is not because of some underlying medical condition but instead, it is because of the amount of stress that they are under or the way that they treat their body.

Make sure that you are drinking enough water, getting the exercise that your body needs, eating healthy meals, dealing with the stress that you are under, and allowing yourself time to relax every single day.

Only then are you going to find that your body is going to be able to truly rest and you are going to get the sleep that you need.

Of course, if all of this fails, going to your doctor and discussing the problem with them is always an option. It should not be the first option though. Taking medication in order to treat something that can be treated with lifestyle changes should never be the first option. Medications come with side effects; lifestyle changes do not.

Be willing to put in the work, and before you know it, you will be sleeping better than you have ever slept before.